All Life Is In The Blood

All Life Is In The Blood

*A medical perspective of
the blood of Christ.*

Ike Pauli, MD.

Xulon Press
2301 Lucien Way #415
Maitland, FL 32751
407.339.4217
www.xulonpress.com

Printed in the United States of America.

ISBN-13: 978-1-54565-955-7

For the life of the flesh *is* in the blood, and I have given it to you upon the altar to make atonement for your souls; for it *is* the blood *that* makes atonement for the soul.

—Leviticus 17:11, NKJV

DEDICATION

Memories take me back to a small, red-brick church in San Antonio, Texas, on Nacogdoches Road. I remember my mother trying to drag me to Sunday school when I would rather go to the church service. The sermons still echo in my mind—"Anything is possible with God (Luke 18:27 NKJV)." "All things are possible to them who believe (Mark 9:23)."

I can still remember walking out of the church at the end of the service as the pastor shook my hand and patted my head. This pastor of my childhood was larger than life. After I returned to the church as a teenager, his sermons gave me encouragement, direction, and carried me through the darkest times of my life. "You can do all things through Christ who strengthens you (Phil. 4:13)." "Seek first the kingdom of God and His righteousness, and all these things shall be added to you (Matt. 6:33)." Always quoting the scriptures and "Truth is not what I say it is, Truth is not what you say it is, Truth is what God's Word says it is."

As I embarked upon college, medical school, and residency, his wisdom, counsel, blessings, and prayers encouraged me to reach beyond what the world told me so many times that I could not do. During times when I was exhausted and at the end of my rope, I would hear his voice in a sermon, "If you are at the end of your rope . . . jerk a knot in it and hang on! . . . They that endure to the end shall be saved (Matt. 24:13)." "God is still on His throne and everything is going to be alright! and Be faithful until death, and I will give you the crown of life (Rev. 2:10)."

Yes, I have been saved by the blood of Christ, but I have been discipled by my pastor. The pastor of my youth is my pastor today, and to me, he is still larger than life—Rev. John C. Hagee, Ed.

To my mother, who wrote the letter that resulted in my salvation. To my father, who provided much-needed stability during my chaotic childhood.

To my beautiful and wonderful wife of over thirty years, Vicki, who has stood beside me and supported me through my career and ministry. We have shared and sacrificed everything together. I would choose no other with whom to take this incredible journey.

To my precious daughter, Paisley, who has put up with her daddy working countless hours. You have given up much of your daddy so that thousands of other children might have a better chance at life. I will never forget all of the nights you tried to wait up, only to have me rock you to sleep. All of my love and devotion *forever*.

To my Lord and Savior, Jesus the Christ, who saved and changed a lonely, broken, and worthless child and made him a man. All that I am that is decent, good, and of worth is due to the everlasting grace of God. May all praise, glory, and honor be given to Him.

ACKNOWLEDGMENTS

One of the greatest difficulties of medical school is the volume of information that one has to learn. Another of the great difficulties is learning the medical language or jargon that we all have to assimilate to communicate effectively in our profession. What we never really learn in school is the ability to communicate that language with the layman or general public. Such has been the most difficult part of writing this book—communicating my revelations on paper for all to understand yet maintaining realism and credibility.

Thank you, the love of my life, Vicki, for pushing me to complete and make this manuscript more readable. Also, all my gratitude for allowing me the time to finish this project, as our time is something that is extremely limited.

A special thanks to a dear friend, Theresa Lockwood, for her professional expertise in the initial editing of this manuscript. She helped me immensely in restructuring and organizing this enormous project.

To Nana, Mrs. Diana Hagee, First Lady of Cornerstone, who has watched over and cared for me and my family for years. Thank you for your time and help in the final edits and

All Life Is In The Blood

advice for several chapters in this manuscript. Out of all the things you do, you don't have the time to help—but you made the time, and I am eternally grateful.

Finally, my enduring gratitude to Dr. Scott Farhart, MD for coaching me in the final edits of *All Life Is In The Blood*. He has always been a medical mentor, an amazing friend of thirty years, and an elder brother in Christ. Thank you for everything you have done for me, my family, and my career.

x

Table of Contents

A PHYSICIAN'S CONFESSION

Medical school, an experience riddled with irony. It is a place that one learns to preserve life by initially studying death. The first semester of medical school is the tremendous hurdle that separates the serious adventurer from those who are just there for the ride. It is an adventure that can be long, tiring, brutal, and yet has more thrills than the fastest roller coaster in America. The first stop is always Gross Anatomy. For most, Gross Anatomy is their first experience with death. I have often wondered why a profession that is dedicated to the provision of life starts its education by studying a corpse.

It doesn't take a doctor to realize that I am speaking of the cadavers that are donated for science. That first day, I found myself staring at the back of what was once a living, breathing, human being with a soul, personality, thoughts, and dreams. It didn't take long, however, before I began to focus on the task of learning my first day's material in an effort to block out the sentimental. (Now, as a seasoned physician with the experiences that I have had with death, I wish that I had stood back a little longer.) In spite of it all, that day, a new world began to unfold within this marvelous body.

An incredible miracle began to unfold beneath the skin of this shell of a human being. It is a miracle in the truest sense. I honestly believe, if left to chance alone, every human being would have major deformities, diseases, and would probably die in early infancy. With the millions of complex reactions, interactions, and metabolic processes within the human body occurring constantly in perfect synchrony, if left to chance alone, would seemingly dictate disaster. Through the next several weeks, I discovered origins and insertions of muscles, complex internets of nerves, and organized pipelines of arteries and veins.

Later in this class, I discovered amazing organs, tissues, and systems that are complex and astonishing. The heart, for example, is one of the most wonderful organs in the body. Beating a hundred times per minute, it would beat 144,000 times per day, and 52,560,000 times per year. It may beat perfectly sixty to one hundred times per minute for seventy-five years; yet if flawless function is not maintained, and a few beats missed, blood flow stops, and death occurs.

The brain, which is the central processing unit for almost every bodily function, seems most complex. It is the processor for approximately fifty miles of nerves reaching every tissue and providing nearly instantaneous information exchange. The brain is the most advanced central processor and hard drive and is capable of holding hundreds of terabytes of information. It filters, compiles, sorts, learns, processes, and stores more information in a day than the best computers can in years.

I found the kidneys to be remarkable organs that selectively filter and reabsorb nutrients, electrolytes, and wastes. Kidneys also regulate the blood pressure, acidity, osmolarity (a measure of concentration), and even the number of red blood cells in the body. They are one of the most unusual organs that cannot be duplicated, even with today's technology. In the halls of medicine, it is said the dumbest kidney is smarter than the most intelligent intern.

As my time in medical school advanced, I learned more and more about the blood. As I trained, I found that most diseases are diagnosed by examining the blood, and most medical treatments take place through the blood. I experienced that taking a sample of blood will represent a sample of the body's functions and dysfunctions. It is a wondrous substance that contains all the healing properties of the body, provides protection for the body, transports waste for and cleanses the body, and unites every organ and tissue together. Yes, underneath the skin lies untold and countless wonders designed by a great architect that, in many ways, can only be studied through the blood and death of another.

In medicine, we face life and death decisions daily. What may seem a simple illness could end in disaster if the physician's skills are not kept sharpened and alert. To many doctors, death has become an adversary. It can be an adversary so guile and cunning that we spend hundreds of thousands of dollars and decades of training trying to defeat it. Ironically, with each tragic death, we learn something a little more about the disease we fight—and ourselves.

Such is Christianity: we *must face death* before we can fully understand the miracle of eternal life. The believer must confront and ponder his own mortality through the death of another, that is, Jesus the Christ. For centuries, Jewish priests would perform sacrifices to obtain forgiveness of sins, so the people would live. This sacrifice would take the place of the people and assume the judgment and penalty of death. Somehow, it is invariably true that in order to experience life, one must ultimately experience death. Could it be that life cannot be understood without experiencing death?

I have found it true in medicine, and I *know* it to be true of Christianity.

> Therefore, we were buried with Him through baptism into death, that just as Christ was raised from the dead by the glory of the Father, even so we also should walk in newness of life. For if we have been united together in the likeness of His death, certainly we also shall be in the likeness of His resurrection, knowing this, that the body of sin might be done away with, that we should no longer be slaves of sin. For he who has died has been freed from sin. (Rom. 6:4–7 NKJV)

The fact is irrefutable—the key to understanding the practice of medicine is to understand the structure and function of the human body, the environment in which it lives, and the pathology its adversaries create. The key to understanding the Christian faith is understanding the necessity of Christ's virgin birth as a divine, human infant, His blood shed on the cross, His death as a man, and His glorious resurrection (1 Cor. 15:3–14). As a physician, I do not hold the keys to the great adversary of death. However, as a Christian physician, I do know of *One* who does hold the keys to death, hell, and the grave (Rev. 1:18). In this confidence, I know that death is not the undefeated adversary. Although physicians have been empowered to *treat* some illness, the Great Physician, because of His shed blood and resurrection, has been empowered to *heal* all illness.

Within this text, I have shared my experiences of both the lives and tragic deaths of those whom I have cared for during my training and practice. Names have not been used; gender and age have been arbitrarily assigned to protect patient privacy. I offer these personal encounters as a tribute to and lasting memory of those who have lost their lives to disease— the result of sin entering the world, thus imparting to me the knowledge of treating those diseases and the revelation of the powerful role the blood plays both medically and spiritually. Just as within the human body dwells countless secrets, so also the blood of Jesus holds countless miracles for those who dare to accept and are covered by His blood.

These experiences will provide greater understanding that: *All Life Is in the Blood.*

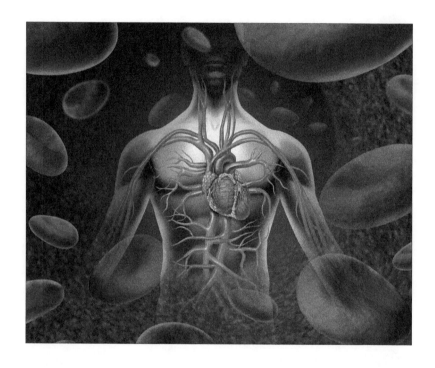

THE BLOOD OF ANOTHER MAN

I t was my third year in medical school, and I was on call rotating through the hematology unit at the local Veteran's Hospital. I was nearing the end of my third year, so I felt that I was prepared for just about anything. I was wrong; it proved to be a night I will never forget.

I was caring for a patient who was a thirty-year-old white male who had chronic myelogenous leukemia (CML). He had a genetic mutation that caused this disease to be very resistant to conventional therapy. Having previously been treated with a bone marrow transplant, he relapsed after only a short remission in full blast crisis (an overwhelming explosion of malignant cancer cells).

In an effort to control my patient's raging cancer, he was re-treated with chemotherapy while awaiting a matched, unrelated donor for his second bone marrow transplant. The toxicity of this last onslaught of chemotherapy, however, wiped out what was left of his bone marrow (the cells inside of the bones where all blood cell production takes place). As a result, he was receiving daily transfusions of blood products including red blood cells (cells that carry oxygen) and platelets (cells that are responsible for clotting) to sustain his life. By this time, my patient was becoming more and more ill, refusing to eat, and wasting away. In spite of everything, I watched his faithful wife, stay by his side caring for him, day in and day out.

The day came all too quickly when we could no longer keep up with the depletion of his platelets, and my patient began to bleed. At first, it was a few simple nosebleeds, but by night's end, it was a deadly pulmonary hemorrhage (blood filling the lungs). Once my patient started retching and vomiting blood, we knew that it wouldn't be long before he would sustain acute pulmonary hemorrhage, leaving him to drown in his own blood.

That night, it happened. I ran into the room amidst cries of help to a nightmare of blood pooled on the floor. I looked down in horror to see a bedpan nearly full of vomited blood as his wife screamed for my help. I watched him gasping for air, coughing, and twisting his body in contorted positions. Immediately, we made attempts to secure his airway, which could only be accomplished by inserting a breathing tube down his windpipe.

The crash cart was brought out as the critical care team arrived to help with the endotracheal intubation in a last effort to save my patient's life. As we attempted to intubate him, bullets of blood were shooting across the room, some even hitting the ceiling. Futile attempts were made by the nursing staff to shield us from the bullets of blood with gowns and face shields. However, by the time we transported him to the medical intensive care unit (MICU) and placed him on the ventilator, he had lost too much blood and too much blood was filling his lungs.

After we made the transfer, (in spite of the paper gowns and face shields that the nurses placed on me while I was caring for him) I looked down at my scrubs, wiped my face, and realized that I was covered in blood—and it wasn't my own.

By then it was 2:00 a.m., and I had been at the hospital for nearly eighteen hours, my patient was dying, and I was covered in his blood—not a day that I was prepared for. After such an exhausting night, my senior residents felt sorry for me and sent me home, a rare thing for a medical student to be able to go home on a call night. Once home, I went straight into the shower to find some way to wash away the trauma of the day. As I was standing in the warm water, scrubbing the remaining blood from my body, a panorama of thoughts and memories flooded my mind amidst the steam billowing through the room.

My mind began recalling the events of the evening, including the horror etched on the face of my patient and the faces of my colleagues working through this disaster. I remembered the face full of tears from his brokenhearted wife as she was told that her husband was dying. And as I lay my head against the cold shower tile with the hot water beating down my back, I began to pray for my patient, his wife, and my ability to cope with what I had just experienced. It was one of the longest showers of my life. Somehow, I was hoping the shower would wash the night's events away altogether.

Later, as I lay in my bed, my body exhausted, my tired eyes fixed on the ceiling in the surrounding darkness, an incredible thought pierced my soul. Not only had I been covered in blood, but I had been covered with the blood—of another man. I knew then, my life would never be the same. By the time I had this realization though, my patient had taken his last breath, perishing due to acute pulmonary hemorrhage. Ironically, he had drowned in the very thing that gave him life.

The more I pondered the thought, the more real it became. All life is in the blood, but in a way, I had not yet connected as a future physician. How profound! How incredible! I don't think I fully understood until that moment, though I had known the biblical principle for over a decade. Now, having completed my training as a physician, I have decided to share with others my experiences and understanding, relating the incredible truths about the blood that flows through our veins and the profound parallels with the shed blood of Jesus Christ.

The blood within our bodies has a specific identity and has amazing healing properties. The blood also plays important roles in forgiveness and cleansing the body. The blood provides protection against infection, unites the entire body, and is the sole transport of energy and waste. These same functions are all spiritually performed by Jesus Christ's blood that was shed on the cross. I know, beyond a shadow of a doubt, that this revelation will change your life if you take time to understand these truths and apply them to your life. For I can assure you, once you have been covered by the blood of another Man—your life will never be the same because all life is in the blood.

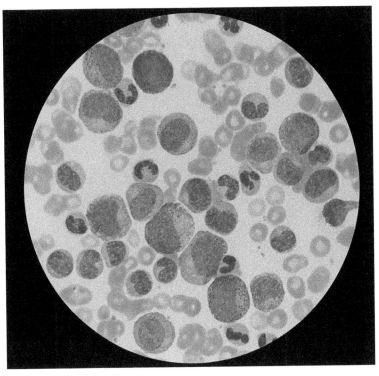

Microscopic view of blood sample with Chronic Myelogenous Leukemia

Chapter One

LIVING WITH BLOOD

I will begin our journey together with a few brief excerpts of my life. While these stories may seem melodramatic, I assure you they are true. These accounts are intended to highlight some life challenges that drove me to the cross, causing me to experience the life-changing power of the blood of Christ.

I have waited for some time to tell my story because the Fifth Commandment is precious to me, and I, in no way, wish to dishonor my parents or their memory. However, some of my stories must be told, so others can find the courage to reach beyond their past and avoid being a mere statistic like so many other victims. I share these testimonies as heartfelt offerings substantiating the power of God in my life, truly defying the challenges and difficulties of this world.

When I was around five years of age, I was awakened from a deep sleep by a flurry of curse words, shouting, blaring music, and loud banging. I remember, quite vividly, my mother dragging me from my bedroom with the smell of alcohol on her breath, half-dressed, and with blood dripping from her face and arms. It seemed like everyone in the house was shouting and as confused as I was.

I remember being horribly terrified as my mother had my arm in one hand and a silver snub-nosed .38 revolver in the other. I recall being dragged out of the house and my stepfather chasing my mother and me several times around the car that was parked in the driveway. This man, who was one of many stepfathers I would eventually have, was just as bloody as my mother was.

As I learned later, an "innocent" party with a "few drinks" escalated into an "innocent" strip tease which then erupted into a jealous bloody brawl, apparently after my stepfather touched another woman in an inappropriate way. I do not remember much else from that evening other than the blinking lights of police cars. However, the most piercing and sustaining memory of that night was the stench of the mixture of blood and alcohol.

We did not live in that house much longer after that frightful altercation. No one died that night except many friendships and a little piece of me. As the wee hours of the night concluded, I finally fell back to sleep in the dark, in my tears, scared and all alone.

As a child, I often wished that dark day never happened because it was a cruel omen of years to come. It was also my first introduction to my mother's angry personality brought out by alcohol, though it had been in my family for generations.

My grandparents entered Texas from the Oklahoma Reservation, so my mother was fully Cherokee in the truest sense. I also recall that my grandfather struggled with a bad temper and alcohol abuse in his younger years and the apple did not fall from the tree when it came to my mother. The stereotype and folklore of the effects of alcohol on the Native American is often depicted in old movies and books. However, it was not folklore in my family—the drinkers got mean . . . just plain mean.

Once again, when I was about ten, I was awakened from sleep hearing, "Shhhhhhh! Do not move! Come with me quick! I have snakes all over me . . . come help me get them off!"

I was exceedingly frightened as the nauseating smell of alcohol permeated the dark room. "Let's go to the bathroom and shake them off. . . . I think I've been bitten!" my mother said, as we staggered to the bathroom. Once there, in full light, I pulled a few leaves off her clothes and out of her hair and asked where she had been. I was trembling and frightened out of my mind. "I'm hiding from them, so they won't get me," she said.

"Who?" I asked.

"Them," she replied as she dragged me outside in the cold and bitter nighttime air. I clung to a blanket I'd taken from my room, and I dragged it on the dirty ground behind me as we ran and hid under a large twenty-foot diameter bush that I often played underneath during the day. It was the first time I had been in there at night, and it was creepy. It was even more scary hiding from someone created by my mother's inebriated mind.

As I shivered in the cold, I could see the vapor generated by my breathing. We stayed out there for most of the night until I talked her into going back inside and letting me go back to bed. After I went to my room, my mother continued to roam the house. Even though I knew the snakes were imaginary, I was still haunted by the fear. What was a ten-year-old to think? After all, it was somewhat weird, pulling imaginary snakes off my mother in the middle of the night. I finally fell back to sleep in the dark, in my tears, scared and all alone.

Morning finally came, and we began to look for hidden keys, glasses, and several other items my mother hid while she was roaming the house. It took us a week to find everything she hid from her demons that night, and later, we even had a few good laughs about it. It was also my first experience with the paranoid personality that manifested within my mother through the effects of alcohol. It was the first but not the last time I met that personality. Sadly, I grew accustomed to meeting that person during a hard drunk. It was uncanny how paranoid she got when under the influence of alcohol.

As a child though, I did not have the knowledge, education, maturity, or insight to understand the things that were happening. It was always so very frightening. Ironically, we would always laugh the next day as we shared stories of the crazy things she would do and where she would hide things. I guess it was a way of easing the embarrassment, the confusion and the terror of the previous night. It must be a cold, frightening reality to wake up knowing one has lost total control, as well as a day or a week of memories. Nevertheless, these horrible episodes were not enough to curb or break her addiction to alcohol.

My mother's sixth marriage almost destroyed me emotionally. I cannot remember a time for over ten years when my mother and stepfather were ever without a beer in their hand

and were not in some sort of confrontation. The house, on occasion, would reek of old beer cans. The cars stank even worse due to the Texas heat further fermenting half-empty old beer cans left rolling around on the floor.

Another experience with the abusive personality manifested by alcohol occurred when I was eight years old. I remember only parts of this specific night and believe my mind has blocked out much of it due to its psychological trauma. As I lay in bed, I heard screaming between my mother and stepfather. I came out of my room and saw my stepfather striking my mother while she screamed. She was fighting back to no avail. Her face was bloody, and her shirt was torn and bloodstained. Once again, the stench of alcohol permeated the room.

I did not know what to do—I was so angry at that moment that I ran and got a baseball bat and began to hit him. I was so filled with hate that I hoped I had killed him—a horrible thought from an eight-year-old child. Later that night, I remember twisting his sunglasses into a ball of contorted metal. I honestly do not recollect what happened to the remainder of the night other than it was then that I learned to hate.

As I have looked back, I realized hatred is a sad and frightening emotion for a child to carry. Hate only builds over time and is more destructive than a nuclear weapon. It is a negative feeling that stores a lot of destructive energy producing long-lasting effects.

Another memory, at ten years of age, was when life abruptly changed. The day had started out great and quickly turned sour. We were running errands, laughing, and having fun, but with a few misspoken words everything flipped in a heartbeat. I had learned all too well that a good day could go bad very quickly in my family. As a pediatrician now, I look back and can understand why I always had stomachaches when visiting my mother; it was caused by emotional stress. I see this often in children in my practice as well. Somehow, the fun turned bitter as my mother began yelling and screaming at my stepfather and then tried to jump out of the car while we were going thirty miles an hour in the middle of traffic.

I remember my stepfather stopping the car and my mother bouncing out of the car like a rubber ball. We managed to drag her back into the car without being hit by traffic. The remainder of the trip was full of screaming, slapping, and fists flying the whole way home. This was not anything new, but what happened next was the last straw for my young mind. As we were getting out of the car, upon reaching the house, my mother grabbed a wine bottle that was in the car and broke it, holding the neck of it like a knife at my stepfather. The next thing I knew, my mother and stepfather were rolling around on the ground trying to cut each other into a bloody mess.

I was so scared I did not know what to do, and just at that moment, by God's timing and grace, my father "happened" to call. I answered the phone we had in the back and told him what was happening, and he rushed over. By the time my father arrived, my mother had gone inside the house and locked herself in the bathroom. We heard her popping pill bottles, so my father kicked the door down and ran in and thwarted her efforts to end her life.

I told my father that I could not take it any longer. That was the last day I lived with my mother. By the following week, he pulled up in his truck and moved my things out. As I was walking out of the house, my mom's last words to me were, "How could you do this to me?" She actually thought that I was rejecting her—probably because she could not remember what happened that day. Maybe she just could not deal with the reality of the recent events and accept the responsibility for her actions.

I still remember the expression on her face; it was almost hateful. Somehow, as a child, she made me feel that the whole thing was my fault. These were just a few of my experiences with the personalities of rage, violence, embarrassment, rejection, and a broken heart brought about by an addiction to alcohol.

While I lived with my mother, I remember coming home on several occasions to an empty house. I would step over a spilled bottle of pills that I would clean up. Hours later, I would receive a call saying my mom was in the hospital and that someone would be home soon to make sure I was all right. Whoever came would disappear again, leaving me frightened and all alone. No one ever told me why, but even at a young age I knew that for some reason my mother tried to take her life.

Later, even though I moved in with my father, weekend visitations became a foreboding nightmare. I love my parents very much, but as a child I had a hard time dealing with the emotional roller coaster ride. Some days were awesome as my mom was always the life of the party. Other days were filled with the horrors I have described.

7

I was told I was loved but always wondered how this could be if I was treated in this way. How could my mother choose to stay with any of my stepfathers even though they treated her and me like that? When my mom did not have a man in her life, I was the center of her soul. When someone else showed up, I felt I was second fiddle. I had come to the realization that she loved them more and that I would always be second, or third, behind any other man and a bottle of wine.

I learned the harsh reality of being a stepchild, seemingly always there waiting to pick up any of the scraps, leftover attention, or love. I learned early about the suicidal personality and the pain of rejection that a person under the influence of alcohol can bring.

Well, obviously that marriage failed — again. The next marriage, my new stepfather took my mother to Thailand, Brazil, Houston, South Texas, and Oklahoma. By this time, I had learned to survive without my mother. I had become quite independent, walled off, and used to my mother not being around. Even though it hurt, by age of fifteen, I learned not to cry when my mother would leave for months or years at a time.

My next stepfather, however, seemed to be a step up from some of the others, as in his own way, he actually seemed to care. He would let me work for him during my summer and winter vacations. Therefore, I would travel to where he and my mother were to visit, work, and make money for tuition. Nevertheless, it was still the same song, second verse — he too was an abusive alcoholic.

However, by this time something very significant had happened in my life; I had a relationship with Christ. This transformation helped me to overcome the rejections of my past—or so I thought.

I was eighteen when I went to Zapata, near Laredo in South Texas to visit Mom and to work on another oil rig. I would roughneck between college semesters and during the summers because it was great money, even though it was hard, dangerous work. One night after a twelve-hour shift, I returned home to an empty trailer house. After fixing dinner, I sat down to eat, and began to pray as I knew something was wrong since no one was at home. I had the same odd feeling I had as a child when I would come home and find pills scattered on the floor.

A few hours later, the phone rang and a trembling voice rattled through the phone. "Ike, I am at a hotel, and I just wanted to let you know that I am going to end my life . . . but I also wanted to let you know that I love you." I tried talking to my mother and find out where she was, but she started screaming at me, laying the blame on me that I was the cause to her problem; then all I heard was a click and a dial tone. I ran out of the house and frantically drove all over Laredo searching for her car in parking lots, all the while not knowing if this time she was serious or just drunk and looking for attention.

I returned to the trailer at midnight and as I walked through the door, I got a call from the hospital informing me that my mother was being discharged. I picked up one of her friends and we immediately drove to the hospital. As she staggered out of the emergency room, she shoved a bloody Bible in my hands and told me that she marked pages with her blood on the passages she wanted me to read and then said, "You will understand."

I looked at her—her makeup was smeared from crying, clothes were bloodstained and disheveled, and sutures marked the slits she had made to both of her wrists. Once again, that familiar smell of alcohol and blood saturated the air around her. It almost made me sick. Yet, when I tried to hug her knowing she was in pain, she pushed me away and told me it was my fault. These words were not new to me—I had heard them many times before.

Eventually, we got her to bed, and I stayed up most of the night making sure she didn't attempt to slip out and try to take her life again before she sobered up. I found out later that she had bought a knife from someone on the street, went into her hotel room, and used it to slit her wrists. However, just after she did it the fire department broke the door down to the hotel room and rescued her before she bled to death. Apparently, the man who sold her the knife realized what she was going to do and called 911.

What kind of warped, inebriated mind would do that to themselves and then blame their own child—not just attempt suicide but also blame it on her only son? Could the guilt and rejection of my leaving her home eight years prior still be driving her self-destructive behavior?

By God's grace, I had matured in my relationship with Christ enough to know it was not my fault, but the pain of hearing her words of blame still cut to my core. I thank the Lord that by that time I had been taught the Word of God for three years and knew that the blood she had spilled meant nothing. The only blood I needed to be concerned with was the blood of Jesus Christ. His blood forgave me. His blood redeemed me, and it was His blood that would heal me from my past. I clung to the fact that Christ loved me enough that He gave His life for mine. Knowing the scripture, "When my father and my mother forsake me, then the Lord will take care of me (Ps. 27:10 NKJV)." I found consolation in who I had become.

I can think of no better way to begin this book than with my personal testimony. How could I substantiate my convictions without providing a personal endorsement? How does one choose a new car or even what movies to see or restaurant to try? The choice is made, in part, by the testimonials and recommendation of others. How do people judge a diet plan? They are convinced through testimonials and seeing before and after pictures, which tell the story.

In this light, the previous few of many excerpts from my life are written not to cause you to sympathize but to help you understand just how powerful the grace of God and the blood of Christ can be. In spite of all the emotional turmoil and anguish my experiences caused, they are nevertheless a part of my life and who I am. When I look at my past, I honestly do not regret what happened because I know God would not let me go through more than I could endure. He has and will continue to use my experiences for His glory.

Bitterness, fear, and regret have no place within me as all of my hurt, pain, and rejection drove me to the cross that

11

redeemed me from my past. And because of that gift, I embrace every experience. Overcoming the garbage in my past is a testimony of the power of the blood of Christ in forgiveness, unity, self-identity, healing, and life itself! Let me boldly proclaim that I have undergone the transforming power of the Gospel of Jesus Christ. What is so miraculous is that I have overcome my negative experiences and have used them to continue to better myself as well as making them into tools to help others.

- Through the blood of Christ, I have been cleansed.
- Through the blood of Christ, I have been healed and restored.
- Through the blood of Christ, I have overcome the destruction of my past.
- Through the blood of Christ, I have protection from disease, bitter memories, rejection, guilt, and inadequacy.
- It is through the blood of Christ that I have forgiveness for my emotions, past actions, hatred, bitterness, and fear.
- It is through the blood of Christ that I have identity as a joint heir in Christ Jesus and heir to the promises of Abraham.
- It is through the blood of Christ that I have harmony, unity, and reconciliation with God, man, and self.

I am now driven to accomplish and succeed in life not with the purpose to gain the approval of my mother, father, wife, or child, but rather to show the world the high calling in Christ Jesus. I am by no means perfect, never have been, and never will be in this life—just ask my wife. I am still a work in progress.

Nevertheless, you must recognize that if someone with my background can rise above life's heartbreaks, anyone can. If God can work miracles in my life, He can work miracles in anyone's life. If I can conquer my past hurts, insecurities, rejections, fears, and failures, anyone can—but only through the blood of Jesus Christ.

I recently had the honor of giving my testimony before my Cornerstone Church family. Some came to me and said, "I'm really sorry you had to go through that." Once again, my reply was, "I'm not! It drove me to the cross. It has given me a powerful testimony for Christ." Proof of the change in my life lies in the fact that my daughter, who is now in her twenties, and is herself in medical school, has never known the sting of alcohol addiction. The curse has been broken through the blood of Jesus Christ!

Though she has experienced some rejection from her grandmother, we, her parents, have never abused, neglected, or abandoned her. She has never been left alone, afraid, or crying into the dark night. She has known the Lord early in life and has served the Lord for years. She has a loving family and wants for nothing.

We have an amazing relationship full of love, trust, and respect. And now I even get to be a medical mentor to her budding career! Only Christ can do that! The curse of generations of alcoholism, divorce, and all of the diseased emotions and personalities of the past has been broken. What was meant for evil, God has made it for the good (Gen. 50:20).

My healing was so complete I have never been to or needed a counselor, psychologist, or psychiatrist. I have never been on any medications for depression, anxiety, or any other mental illness. I have no addictions; have never been drunk or high on drugs a day in my life because of the power of the blood of Jesus Christ. The buck stopped there—at His cross—the curse was broken. The generational bondage was shattered at the cross of Christ through the shedding of His innocent blood.

Are you broken, addicted to some vice, emotion, or illness? Are you rejected, alone, isolated, and feel abandoned by those closest to you? Keep reading! Find out just how powerful the blood of Christ can be!

A profound example happened the other day when my daughter was at our church leadership training. They asked that each person give their personal testimony. Her testimony was rather simple, "I was born at the church, saved at the church, baptized in the church, grew up in the church, and all I have ever known is a godly home."

When asked, "What, no alcohol, no drug addiction, no divorce, no abuse or neglect?" My daughter simply replied, "My father endured and overcame all of that so I didn't have to." She later told me, "You could have heard a pin drop in the room after that." What more needs to be said? Generations of these diseases have been broken, once and for all. All to God's glory.

The last point I want to drive home is that blood and alcohol *do not* mix, not in the chemical sense, of course, but definitely not in the physical, mental, emotional, and spiritual sense. My mom attended church while still having a problem with alcohol. No one knew the problems we had at home except the neighbors. I have prayed with countless children and adults at church, who come forward for prayer claiming their father, mother, or spouse is abusive and/or alcoholic.

I know abuse is in the world and in the church. Therefore, I conclude this chapter by standing on my soapbox for a reason: *drug and alcohol addiction impairs*. Physicians know that it has been proven time and time again that the physical reaction response is adversely affected by even one glass of wine, beer, or similar alcoholic beverage. Alcohol consumption impairs judgment, impulse control, and just about every higher-level brain function. Alcohol can also cause severe birth defects in children born to mothers who drink while pregnant. Even one to two glasses per day is enough to cause a condition known as fetal alcohol syndrome.

As a pediatrician, I am aware of the growing problem of teenage alcohol and drug abuse. With the addition of "girly drinks" (sweet alcoholic beverages), we are witnessing a huge spike in the use and misuse of alcohol among teens. Lest I sound legalistic, I will be the first to admit, however, that alcohol is not evil (Rom. 14:17). Jesus himself drank wine and He will again in heaven (Matt. 26:29). It is the *intent* of the consumption, the *need* for consumption, and the *amount* of consumption of the alcohol that is at issue. The Word of God clearly states to be sober-minded (Titus 1:8; 2:6). It also states it is wise to abstain from strong drink (Prov. 20:1). Finally, it calls for all believers to do all things in moderation (1 Cor. 9:25). Why?

Alcohol and many other drugs are physically and psychologically addictive substances. Alcohol is a drug. It even has a chemical structure (CH_3CH_2OH or ETOH). Surprised? This compound is a chemical that produces physiologic effects within the body and mind—quite simply, it is a drug. Just as it has the ability to depress anxiety and remove inhibitions, it has the same ability to produce dependence. In particular, if a person has an addictive personality, alcohol has a greater physiological and psychological effect and therefore creates a greater chance of dependence.

Some may use alcohol because its effects suppress their fears and anxieties for the trials of life. Others may use it to forget past hurts. It is important to remember to stay sober-minded. While alcohol may help one relax, it can also worsen depression. While it may help one forget, it may also cause dependence. While it may help with anxiety, it may make one less sensitive to the needs of those who are dependent, like a child or spouse.

In addition, alcohol consumption is associated with multiple deaths in auto accidents, numerous abusive relationships, and considerable detrimental effects on one's health, job performance, and mood. I could go on for hours proclaiming the detrimental effects of alcohol from a medical perspective. The bottom line is if you drink, do so in moderation. If you cannot limit your intake sensibly, then do not drink alcohol at all.

I plead with you—do not destroy your life, your spouse's life, or your children's lives. Many times, while visiting my mother in the hospital because of the complications associated with her drinking, physicians would take me to the side and counsel me about the negative side effects of alcohol. They were well-meaning in explaining to me the increased inherited risk I would have for being an alcoholic if I chose to drink. What they did not know was that I was embarrassed because, by then, I had already chosen not to drink. Nevertheless, I would thank them for their counsel and smile, knowing they did not want what was happening to her to become my lot.

I remember spending the evening at an aunt's home when I was eight years old. Once again, alcohol seemed to be the foundation of the event. My mother and aunt left to go out for a few hours and came back pretty hammered. My aunt offered for us to stay the night, but Mom would not have it. She said, "We will be fine." Well, Mom could barely walk much less steer the car.

As a result, my mother had me sit between her legs behind the wheel to help steer while she tried to operate the clutch, brake, and gas peddles since I could not reach them. We made it a couple of blocks and had to turn around because Mom could not seem to coordinate the clutch with the stick—go figure. We managed to get back to my aunt's home and sleep for two to three hours, and then she was ready for round two. By then, Mom had sobered up enough to operate the clutch, gas, and stick, while I managed to steer and operate the brake. God only knows how, but we made it home around 3:00 a.m. This is a perfect example of how alcohol impairs sound judgment, and physical and mental performance. You have to agree that something is wrong with this picture—abuse of alcohol destroys.

Jesus told us in the Gospels that, "My yoke is easy and My burden is light (Matt. 11:30)." He also told us that, "I have come that they may have life, and that they may have it more abundantly (John 10:10)." Finally, He wants us to go to Him with our burdens (Matt. 11:28).

If you have to drink alcohol, you have a problem with dependence. If you cannot have fun without it at a party or cannot socialize without it, you may have a problem with insecurity or social phobia. If you need alcohol to relax, you may have a problem with anxiety or depression. If you need it to deal with the problems of life, then you may have poor coping skills or have lost hope for the future. If you need to drink to survive life with a drunk, you may need a new spouse —or at least counseling to save your marriage.

I encourage you to stop fooling yourself. Step into reality and stop making excuses! My mother, bless her soul, made excuses and used alcohol for all the wrong reasons. It destroyed her life and nearly destroyed mine, if it had not been for the intervention of the blood of Christ. She was a highly intelligent, gifted, beautiful, passionate, and liberated woman. Yet she had eight husbands, did not achieve her full potential, nearly destroyed her child, and lived most of her life physically ill and emotionally crippled. It was only in her later years that she was able to honestly admit: "I am so afraid of being alone."

Prescription opiates are at the forefront of the media. They cause a staggering number of addictions and death in the United States every day. Opiate abuse is now so prevalent that it has become a national crisis. Opiates, crystal meth, alcohol, cocaine, heroin, marijuana, and designer drugs are all the same. They are drugs that can result in addiction, dependence, wrecked lives, and eventually death.

While I used my experience with alcoholism to make important points, addiction to these other substances is just as detrimental! Through God's saving grace, my mother is with Jesus today after a life tattered with bad choices. She passed away nearly ten years ago due to renal failure because of years of complications from a liver transplant due to cirrhosis of the liver. Her cirrhosis was caused by a combination of hepatitis and years of alcohol abuse.

My mother died years before she should have, never fulfilling a meaningful relationship with her only son and her only grandchild! Even though alcohol addiction and the sin of abuse robbed me of a normal childhood and a close and fruitful relationship with my mother, I am able to accept God's perfect plan for my life. God took a cascade of devastating circumstances and fashioned a divine plan in me to have a beautiful marriage, to raise an amazing daughter, to bring healing to children through my profession, and to give hope to those who have walked or are walking a similar journey to mine.

Do not let addiction rob you of your life, your health, your marriage, your children, or your sanity. Go to the cross of Christ, not the bottle, not the inhalant, not the syringe, and not the even the prescription. As a *child*, my initial exposure to *blood* was repulsive and frightful. Conversely, my encounter with the *blood of Christ* has given me a life of peace and joy. Such is the purpose of my story and this book in revealing the liberating power of the blood of Christ. I encourage you to read on and see how you, too, can be covered in the blood of Christ instead of being tormented by alcohol, addiction, disease, and regret.

The bottom line is: do not let your blood and alcohol (addiction) be the stench in the nostrils of others, especially your own children.

Chapter Two

YOU MUST BE BORN AGAIN

❮❮ Most assuredly, I say to you, unless one is born of water and the Spirit, he cannot enter the kingdom of God. That which is born of flesh is flesh, and that which is born of the Spirit is spirit (John 3:5–6 NKJV)." For centuries, people have tried to grasp the concept that Jesus presented to the rabbi called Nicodemus. Being born of water was easy to understand; that is the natural birth. Being born of the Spirit was difficult to understand, even for this respected rabbi. After all, how can the carnal mind understand things of the spirit? "Therefore, if anyone is in Christ, he is new creation; old things have passed away; behold, all things have become new (2 Cor. 5:17)." What is this new life? What is this rebirth? What does it have to do with the blood? There are multiple other passages dealing with this basic concept that even the religious fail to completely understand (Rom. 6:1–14; Eph. 2:12–16; 4:22–24).

I have found, through thirteen years of secular higher education, that this new man or new life that is reborn or transformed through the death of Christ and the Spirit of His resurrection is an apparent mystery to the religious (like Nicodemus), the educated, and even to those who have experienced it.

In one of my literature courses in college, I remember a classmate asking in a condescending tone, "And what about this 'born-again Christianity?' I don't understand it . . . it must be some sort of fad." My rather hasty and heated reply in that secular literature classroom came immediately, without thinking. I replied, "I am one of those 'born-again Christians' and have been for over ten years . . . so much for a fad. And it is something that I really don't expect you to understand. You have to be born again."

At that moment the quiet was absolute, and a pin dropping to the floor could be heard. I glanced at my instructor across the room, preparing for battle, curious about her response, only to see her mouth gaping wide open in amazement. The battle was over at that point, and the subject quickly changed. In that light, I truly believe that it is impossible to understand being born again unless it is experienced. In spite of that fact, I think I have some insights that may help the skeptic and the believer understand the necessity and principles behind this transformation and why Jesus used this profound statement to Nicodemus.

I was moonlighting one night in the neonatal intensive care unit (NICU), attempting to earn a little extra cash to offset my meager salary. Immediately after check-out, a two-hour-old baby girl rolled through the door with our transport team. This baby was ashen in color, sedated, and intubated with a breathing tube in her windpipe to help her breathe. I became concerned as I evaluated her because she had a very fast heart rate, poor blood flow, and a very low oxygen level in her blood. In the back of my mind, I couldn't help wondering what her parents must have been feeling. Instead of hearing their doctor congratulating them on the birth of this new beautiful baby girl, he had to explain to them that their new baby was critically ill and might die.

Once we placed her on the ventilator, I realized that she was requiring extremely high levels of oxygen and high ventilator pressures to achieve normal oxygen levels in the blood. Her chest X-ray was normal, but her oxygen levels in her blood were telling us another story. We then did an echocardiogram, trying to determine the reasons for this baby's serious illness. It revealed very high blood pressures in the blood vessels of the lungs. It also showed that the natural hole between the upper chambers of the heart (which is needed while the baby is in the womb) was open, with blood passing freely passing through. In other words, the flow of blood was still similar to that which was in the womb. We call this problem primary pulmonary hypertension (PPHN) with persistent fetal circulation. It is uncommon, but if left untreated, it can be extremely lethal.

We decided to use a new treatment that was considered experimental at that time. It was my first experience with this new therapy delivered through the ventilator called nitric oxide (not the laughing gas many associate with a dentist that is nitrous oxide). In simple terms, it is designed, to lower the blood pressure in the lungs. If this failed it would mean placing this newborn infant on extracorporeal membrane oxygenation (ECMO), which is similar to a heart/lung machine and carried considerable risks. As we dialed up the dosage of this miracle gas, I was amazed. The oxygen requirements immediately reduced, and the flow of blood in the heart and lungs became normal. Over the next few days, we were able to wean her off of this miracle gas and the ventilator as this infant's flow of blood returned to its new normal state. We saved her life.

A fetus, or unborn child, has a completely different circulation of blood than that of the newborn child and adult. Outside of the womb, our heart's circulation is *centered around the lungs* since the lungs are the source of oxygen for the body. Conversely, the fetal circulation of blood is *focused around the placenta*. The blood is circulated from the child to the placenta via three blood vessels in the umbilical cord, delivering wastes and carbon dioxide, while receiving sugars, nutrients, antibodies, and oxygen from the mother. Blood flows from the placenta through the umbilical vein in the umbilical cord and then through a temporary bypass in the liver. Blood then flows to the heart and is guided through the right atrium into the left atrium and then into the left ventricle of the heart, bypassing the lungs. The blood is then pumped by the heart to the baby's body for distribution and eventually back to the placenta for oxygen and nutrition. Some blood may make it into the right atrium and ventricle. This blood is then directed through a temporary duct bypassing the lungs once again since the lungs are not utilized in the womb.

Conversely, with birth, the *entire circulation changes* with a completely different focus. When a baby is born, the placenta is no longer the focus of the circulation. A number of fantastic events occur when the infant takes its first breath and the umbilical cord is clamped. The two ducts in the heart and liver close, the lungs inflate with air, and blood flows through the lungs before being circulated through the body. With the *new focus being the lungs*, there are higher levels of oxygen in the blood. Over the next several weeks after birth, the higher oxygen levels trigger the bone marrow to stop producing fetal red blood cells and start producing adult red blood cells. With everything working perfectly, in a few short months, the adult red blood cells will *completely replace* the fetal red blood cells.

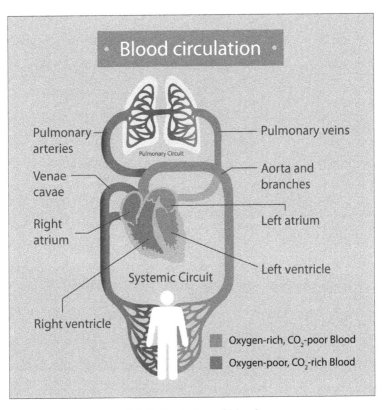

Adult circulation of blood

25

At the time of birth, the *entire circulation changes* to accommodate this new life. Now, if it sounds complicated, that's because it is—yet it takes place spontaneously. The point is not to understand the mechanics, but details were provided for the skeptics. Stop and think about it! God is consistent. He does not create a new life without providing the circulation or empowerment to sustain that life. Also, by creating new life, He does not expect it to hold on to those things maintaining its old existence, circulation, or lifestyles. Just as an infant cannot live with persistent fetal circulation (attached to its umbilical cord and out of the womb), a new believer can't live clinging to his old life—the old life must die. To accomplish this, a *believer's circulation (focus of life)* must change—changing the very essence of his being. The *focus* of his circulation can no longer be himself, but *Jesus Christ*, the one who has delivered him.

Also, just as the infant's fetal red blood cells must die and be removed (being replaced with adult red blood cells) the believer likewise must lay down his life daily, that is, his old life, desires, hopes, and expectations. and allow it to be replaced with a new (reborn) life. Ultimately, and spontaneously, it is a whole shift in focus from one way of life to another without understanding the mechanics. In Romans 6:3–11, Paul reminds us that as we associate with Christ's death, we die to sin, and as such we also share in His resurrection or new life. It is a rebirth as you will recall from the story of Nicodemus; one doesn't go back to where he came from but adapts to and changes his entire way of life.

Many call this process sanctification, which is accomplished only by being transfused by the shed blood of Jesus and being changed daily by His Spirit. "And be renewed in the spirit of your mind, and that you put on the new man which was created according to God, in righteousness and true holiness (Eph. 4:23–24)." "And do not be conformed to this world, but be transformed by the renewing of your mind, that you may prove what is that good and acceptable and perfect will of God (Rom. 12:2)." Just as an infant, when born, must completely separate from its mother to survive, the believer, when reborn, must separate himself from the carnal, the old life, the world, and be transformed by the God who has given that new life.

Medical complications may occur if the umbilical cord is clamped too late, as the infant may receive too many red blood cells and have a complicated transitional period. Complications include low blood sugar, stroke, kidney failure, intestinal ischemia, jaundice, and potential kernicterus (brain damage from extreme jaundice). Thus, a partial, incomplete, or delayed separation will result in death or illness. Likewise, spiritually, an incomplete or delayed transformation of the new believer will result in a crippled unproductive life or a return to the old life.

Let me tell you about this new life from personal experience. As noted before, I grew up in a violent and unpredictable alcoholic home, and I had frequent encounters with the usual situations such an environment creates. Neglect, abandonment, violence, exposure to pornography, attempted suicide, rage, cursing, bloody fights, and gunfire were frequent exposures in my young life.

By the time I was fifteen years old, I was mixed up, without identity, lonely, isolated, weak, vulnerable, bitter, insecure, and without hope. I walked into Cornerstone Church on February 18, 1980. I heard the Gospel of Jesus Christ's birth, death, and resurrection, and I asked Him into my heart and life. I walked out of that church a changed youth, and I have never been the same. My thoughts, actions, deeds, desires, and motivations have all been different since that day. I was never the same; I became a new creature. My new life began, and I was ready to leave my old life behind.

So, Nicodemus, truly you too must be born again—reborn by the power of the shed blood of Jesus the Christ. No, you can't go back where you came from. Old things must pass away, and all things become new. *New life is in the blood.*

Chapter Three

IDENTITY IN THE BLOOD

W hat are the chances that two children in the same family would come down with cancer within six months of one another? The possibility would undoubtedly be close to the same chances of winning the lottery two times in the same year. I experienced this situation in my second year in the hematology-oncology transplant (HOT) unit.

I admitted a fifteen-month-old baby boy with acute lymphocytic leukemia whose older brother was diagnosed with the same illness six months earlier. The cure rate for this disease is approximately eighty to ninety percent, however, this child was sent to us for a bone marrow transplant since his leukemic cell line had a particular genetic abnormality that could not be cured with conventional chemotherapy. What a fate! I don't know how I would handle this happening to my own flesh and blood, but the family of these two patients demonstrated incredible courage, integrity, and unity.

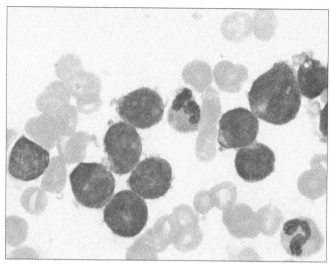

Microscopic view of blood sample with Acute Lymphocytic Leukemia

Bone marrow transplants have saved thousands of lives that would have otherwise succumbed to cancer. It is, however, one of the most grueling and taxing procedures a human being can endure. The words are easy to pronounce, give a hideous vision, and yet mechanically it is quite simple. It begins by intensive chemotherapy with medications that cause vomiting, hair loss, diarrhea, headaches, body aches, blurred vision, itching, shaking, chills, and can make every mucous membrane in a body blister. If you multiply the misery of the flu by fifty, it might just approximate what the patient goes through. The chemicals used are so potent and toxic that special catheters or ports are placed in the larger central veins to dilute them during administration. If infused in a peripheral vein, it would shrivel the vein into a thin rubber band. Likewise, some will easily cause a severe burn or tissue to rot if even contacted with the skin. This induction chemotherapy is intensified and followed by several days of total body irradiation. If the patient has not become incredibly ill yet, just wait. It actually takes several days to see and feel the effects of destroying every rapidly dividing cell in the body. The experience could probably be compared with a tour through the Agent Orange–filled jungles of Vietnam.

After several days in total misery, surviving daily blood draws to ensure that all of the cells in the bone marrow are destroyed, all the body's electrolytes are balanced, and the body's organs are functioning properly, another person's bone marrow is dripped into the recipient's veins. Remarkably, the donor's bone marrow cells find their way to the recipient's bone marrow to begin reproduction. Now the wait begins for the signs of engraftment, where the donor's bone marrow replaces the patient's old marrow and begins to reproduce its new cell lines. It is kind of like a home that has one family replacing another after the former has moved. The wait is hallmarked by more daily blood draws, transfusions, continuous intravenous antibiotic therapy, being locked up in a positive pressure room (sometimes for weeks), and having to experience all sense of touch made through latex gloves and gowns while visitors hide behind paper masks.

Now, take a step back and view this through a child's eyes. Why do I detail the procedure so? To show what this beautiful fifteen-month-old boy had to undergo during this horrid process. He was not capable of understanding why and what was happening to him. There is a lot of science to a bone marrow transplant with millions of complexities involved. This little child, however, had no clue to what was taking place within his body. As the days went by, I walked in each day and watched his smile and laugh become a cry and look of despair. I watched his mouth swell, his airway almost close, his hair fall out, and his skin blister as a result of graft-versus-host disease. This cheerful little child became a miserable little soldier fighting for his life daily, against a foe he could not see.

On another exhausting tour through the HOT unit, I assumed care of a six-year-old girl who had a very aggressive form of acute lymphocytic leukemia. She was treated with the standard regime of chemotherapy but relapsed within two years of her first treatment. She was retreated a second time and relapsed again within one year. She had returned to us for her only hope—a bone marrow transplant. She also had the misfortune of not having a related, fully-matched donor, nor could one be found through the national registries. Tragically, she ran out of time and the closest match was her mother, though not close enough. She went through the same processes, though with a little more intensity due to the high risks of her unmatched transplant. She was a gifted child with a lot of fight.

She endured her transplant and for a while did quite well. Suddenly, however, she became very ill, running fevers, having horrendous diarrhea, difficulty breathing, and a severe skin rash. We knew much of what was happening was due to what we call graft-versus-host disease. It is a disease where her new blood cells were destroying her body because they were recognizing her as foreign in spite of the high doses of steroids and immunosuppressive medicines we were giving her to control this reaction. This insult seemed to be the trigger to a number of events that made her care quite difficult. I spent many hours during the month caring for her and grew to greatly respect anyone who endures such a disease.

Initially, I would walk in to examine her and she would fight me tooth and nail, as she justifiably and quickly learned to fear doctors. As the days passed, however, I watched her and her mother's struggles dwindle. I watched her hair fall out, her lips and skin blister and watched her vomit until she would collapse from exhaustion. She eventually became so ill that her lungs and kidneys began to fail, and I realized that her body was shutting down. It wasn't long before we had to transfer her to the pediatric intensive care unit (PICU). In spite of the best care in the country, a few weeks later she died.

There are a multitude of cells in the body's blood and hosts of complex proteins governing their interactions. There are white blood cells that fight infection and malignancy. There are cells that aid in clotting called platelets and vascular endo-thelium. And there are red blood cells that carry oxygen and carbon dioxide called erythrocytes. All of these cells have incredibly complex functions and highly specific interactions so particular and tailored that, if altered, would most times spell disaster.

Simply, each of the cells in the human body has marker proteins that give it an entirely *unique identity*. These proteins are of primary importance to the cells of the immune system within the blood. They are the means by which the immune system *recognizes itself* from a *foreign invader*. They function similarly to the way in which a mother uses her five senses to distinguish her children from the children next door. I have explained this interaction to my daughter who is in medical school with the following example: If someone was to show up on your doorstep who you did not know, you would obviously not open the door and let them in but try to ascertain who they were through a peephole, window, or speaking through the door. If a good friend comes to the door with a friend and introduces the stranger, you would open the door without hesitation and shake their hand without reservation.

Why is this so important? In order for a bone marrow transplant (as well as many other transplants) to have the best chance of success, as many of the specific marker proteins must match as possible. If the donor bone marrow is not well matched with the recipient, there is a great chance that the transplant will fail, since the donor marrow will attack all of the recipient's cells and kill them in the process called graft-versus-host disease.

In solid organ transplants like kidney transplants, for example, the reverse may happen in which the recipient's immune system would destroy the foreign organ. These interactions and proteins are so important that huge international registries have been set up to locate donors of similar makeup. It is all about *identity*.

There is a complex identity to every cell in the body defined by an individual's exclusive genetic makeup as described above. Half of these proteins or markers are inherited from the mother and half from the father, so parents won't even share the same makeup as their child. Identity is the primary factor between the interactions of the body and the immune system. If the identity is lost or not tightly regulated, diseases like systemic lupus, rheumatic fever, cancer, Kawasaki's, and rheumatoid arthritis will result. Once again, if the identity is not closely matched, then a transplant will be rejected; worse, the transplant (particularly, a bone marrow transplant) may destroy the body (graft-versus-host disease).

Perfect *identity* is found in the *body and blood*. Just as identity is important in the body's own blood, there is an important *identity* found in the *blood of Jesus Christ*. For, those who receive, are washed in, or transfused with the blood of Christ become marked and identified perfectly as His own. There can be no near match or substitute, or else *it will be rejected and die*. Thus, it is only the blood of Christ that is the most basic identifying factor that gives the believer identity with God.

I know what it is like being a stepchild (many times over), and I can guarantee that one who believes in Christ is no longer a stepchild, but an adopted, grafted-in child of the Living God with an eternal marker—the precious blood of Jesus Christ. "Or do you not know that your body is the temple of the Holy Spirit who is in you, whom you have from God, and you are not your own? For you were bought at a price; therefore glorify God in your body and in your spirit, which are God's (1 Cor. 6:19–20)."

Thousands of years ago, the blood of lambs marked the doorposts of those chosen of God as a sign that the Lord would not allow the destroyer to come into their home (Ex. 12:13, 23). The blood was a sign to the Israelites, God, and the destroyer that those behind the door had special *identity* as God's chosen. Today, it is the blood of the Son of the living God that marks the doorposts of our souls. We then become not only God's creation, but God's children marked with a crimson stain that can never be erased, confused, forgotten, or washed away.

> And they sang a new song, saying: "You are worthy to take the scroll, And to open its seals; For You were slain, And have redeemed us to God by *Your blood* out of every tribe and tongue and people and nation, And have made us kings and priests to our God; And we shall reign on the earth." (Rev. 5:9–10, emphasis added)

Scriptural proof of the blood's identity is affirmatively found in a story of two brothers in the beginnings of time itself. In the book of Genesis, chapter four, we find one brother, Abel, who offered a blood offering from the first fruits of his flock which was accepted and pleasing to God. Cain, however, offered an offering from the ground (toils from his labor) and apparently was not his first fruits. This offering was rejected by God. Even after God counseled and exhorted him (fully knowing what he would do) of the dangers of sin, and that it was up to him to master sin, Cain still killed Abel. When God confronted Cain, in spite of his denial, God told

him, "The voice of your *brother's blood* cries
out to Me from the ground (Gen. 4:10)."

God did not say He saw the incident and heard the screams
of his brother (though He obviously did). The blood of Abel
was crying out—uniquely having an intimate identity with
God. Even after Abel's death, his blood was crying out to God
because there is identity in the blood.

Taking the story back to my patients—the fifteen-month-old
baby boy managed to survive this onslaught of his disease and
treatment and accepted his new bone marrow transplant, sup-
plied by his sister, without rejection and minimal graft-versus-host disease. I followed his course through the years and
saw him grow. He was that smiling, happy child once again.
He even grew his hair back. Now, as I look back, it is hard
to believe that a deadly disease that his body could not control once endangered him. By giving him chemotherapy, we
destroyed his disease. By giving him a transplant, in a sense,
we placed within him a new identity and a new chance for
life. He ultimately survived because his body *accepted its new
identity.* Likewise, the cross destroyed our disease and sin, and
Christ's blood gives us new identity as God's very own if we
choose to accept it!

The six-year-old girl that I cared for, however, unfortunately, did not have the same outcome. This was a tragic loss
of life, one I will never forget. (To this day I still see her face
through teary eyes.) But it does bring home the point that what
one receives can give him life or destroy him tragically. The

new graft that she received attacked her body and destroyed her. The new identity she was given destroyed her because *it was not a near match.* This is the same principle in the spiritual life of man. Identifying with any other thing, process, person, religion, or group in an attempt to find inner peace, healing, or fulfillment will result in destruction. It will only consume and envelope the soul with emptiness, darkness, and despair.

True and everlasting identity with God can only be made through the blood of Jesus Christ. Once again, type-specific blood was drawn from the veins of the Son of God Himself, given freely for the wayward soul. Specifically, finding identity in drugs, alcohol, spray cans, cults, gangs, and the occult are sure ways of securing one's destruction because it is not the cure God intended or provided. If you have had an encounter with Christ and have not had a change in identity, certain death will result. Your identity must change by asking Jesus Christ into your heart through His blood and become the "new creature" (2 Cor. 5:17, KJV) God requires.

For the believer who has received Christ and has accepted His blood as atonement, you have a uniqueness and distinctiveness as God's very own. You are defined, marked, and identified as His child with access, claims, and rights to all of His most precious promises. For God provides for, heals, protects, cares for, loves, disciplines, and draws near to His very own. The apostle Paul clearly illustrates this most simple but powerful premise in Ephesians 2:12–13: "that at that time you were without Christ, being aliens from the commonwealth of Israel and strangers from the covenants of promise, having no hope and without God in the world. But now in Christ Jesus you who once were far off have been brought near by the blood of Christ."

You have to understand identity before you can move on. It is the single most important property of the blood of Christ. You must realize who you are in Christ to further your relationship with God. Are you insecure? Then you lack identity. Do you doubt your purpose on this big blue marble? Then you don't really appreciate the calling you have on your life. Do you lack value, not knowing if you really fit in? Then you don't understand the price Christ paid to purchase your life and make you one of his own. You are more loved and precious than you will ever know.

Please take a moment to self-reflect before reading on. Are you insecure? Do you lack faith? Are you wondering who you really are? Have you been searching for something or someone to give you purpose in this life? Then take this moment and pray. "Heavenly Father, I recognize the price your Son Jesus paid for the redemption of my soul. I need your love. I need to truly know who I am. I need a new purpose in my life. So, I receive Him into my life to give me a new identity and make me a new person. I discard my old ways and want to become part of your everlasting family from this day onward."

Surely, if you have received Christ, your individual identity in Him is certain, specific, and recorded for eternity. Take heart! Most assuredly, there is identity in the blood—everlasting, life-giving, *identity in the blood of Christ.*

MOLTEN LIFE

Turning from within the flaming winded burn,

Pressing to the Light whom once it had spurned,

Flowing through ash as fine liquid gold,

Spewing the magma from its blackened soul.

Scorched and heated, seared from within,

Torched and flamed for life again,

Molten, crawling from ashes past,

Born of New Flame, and Life at last.

Compressed from all sides, relentless toil,

Crushed and molded this black cold coal.

Time is burning, while much has passed,

Molding the work of the future at last.

Near completion, compressed, heated, and burned,

This cold lump of coal, in living turn,

A diamond in birth, nearly complete,

Whence the lifeless black dust, born in God's heat.

—Ike Pauli, MD

Chapter Four

FORGIVENESS IN THE BLOOD

I walked through the door of the examining room to see a young thirteen-year-old girl, tall, slender, wasted, and weak. Her eyes were drawn and dark, her body frail. She came in complaining of weakness and feeling tired for the past several months. I knew that this was serious when her mother told me that during their recent trip to Disney World, she could not muster up the energy to make it through the parking lot. At this time her mother was showing signs of anger, resentment, and concern about her daughter's state. She went so far as to make the remark that her daughter had ruined their trip. She was actually wondering if her daughter was faking it or whether she might have some psychological condition. This girl, who was once a star basketball and volleyball player, now couldn't walk across the parking lot without needing a rest. As we talked further, she told me that her hands would turn blue when exposed to cold and that she had lost twenty pounds in one month. Her hands would even become numb and blue simply holding a cool soda can.

As I began to examine her wasted and drawn body, I noted the tight, drawn skin around her fingers, the flaccid weakness of her muscles, and the swollen, tender joints of her hands, arms, and legs. Her weakness was so profound that she was unable to rise to a standing position from sitting without the use of the hands, which is a sign someone with muscular dystrophy might have. The condition she was suffering from was not difficult to diagnose. She was a young lady with a mixed connective tissue disease, having features of dermatomyositis (condition causing inflammation of skin and muscles), rheumatoid arthritis, and scleroderma (condition causing skin, blood vessels, and other tissues to be replaced by scar tissue). It is a debilitating disease that can take a young, healthy child and turn her into an invalid within a matter of months.

That same month, I consulted on a young fifteen-year-old girl who looked like living death. For the past six months, she had been progressively losing over twenty pounds of weight, had weakness, difficulty concentrating, speaking, and involuntary shaking movements. She was unable to make eye contact with me while sitting on the exam table, holding her hands tightly together in her lap in an attempt to restrain her movements. I began to ask her questions and found that this once straight A high school student was giving me slurred, labored answers as one who had sustained a stroke. She was pale, drawn, and had thin brittle hair. She truly looked like someone who had spent years in a concentration camp.

As I examined her, I noted her abnormal tick-like movements. As she grasped my hands, I recognized her milkmaid grip (rhythmic spasms with voluntary squeezing producing a motion similar to that of milking a cow), malar rash (red, butterfly-shaped rash over face), swollen joints, enlarged liver, and profound weakness. This was truly a sick young girl. We hospitalized her immediately, certain her condition was caused by systemic lupus erythematosus, or worse yet, central nervous system lupus.

Her laboratory tests only confirmed our diagnosis. This young lady was placed on the highest dose of steroids I have ever seen used—over a thousand milligrams was infused in her veins each day for three days. To put it into perspective, she was receiving five times the dosage an average child with a severe asthma exacerbation would receive in a day. As the days progressed, I watched her gain weight, increase in strength, and almost smile. Through the next several months as she received her steroid therapy, I kept in contact and watched her make a near-miraculous improvement. I had the greatest privilege to see her smile and laugh once again, the greatest reward of every pediatrician.

The diseases I have described above have a common thread. Somehow, the body's immune system gets activated against its own tissues (autoimmunity) either by a genetic tendency, an environmental trigger (like a virus or chemical), or both. In any event, the body's identity (recall the last chapter on identity) becomes confused, and the immune system begins to attack its body in an unregulated fashion. Depending on the areas of the body affected and means of attack, the individual disease is manifested.

I have seen many of these illnesses, and some can be hideously debilitating. Virtually all of them can ultimately lead to great pain, suffering, and even death. SLE (systemic lupus erythematosus), mixed connective tissue disease, rheumatoid arthritis, rheumatic fever, scleroderma, Grave's disease, Kawasaki's disease, multiple sclerosis, and myasthenia gravis are but a few diseases caused by autoimmunity.

In normal, healthy individuals, the body's immune system protects itself from invading bacteria, viruses, fungi, parasites, and toxins. This protection is rather remarkable and can be quite violent. Fortunately, the immune system normally regulates itself in perfect harmony. If left unregulated, confused, or disrupted, however, these reactions could be quite devastating. So, the body has immune cells, antibodies, and chemicals that both ignite and adjust its inflammatory reactions.

As mentioned earlier, if the suppressive mechanisms do not function properly or the attacking mechanisms are not adequately controlled, self-destruction will occur. In medicine, we attempt to treat these diseases with medications that suppress the immune system in an attempt to halt the destructive forces. Although these medicines quash the self-destructive reactions, they can do so at a great price. Their side effects can be very toxic to other organs, cells, and tissues, leaving the body vulnerable to infection.

Forgiveness is a must for survival, even in the human body. The body naturally balances its identity with its violent tendencies to protect. The body is able to maintain this balance through a series of complex chemical interactions. This equilibrium is a means of forgiveness that the body must have in order to thrive and survive. There can be no harmony, no health, and no life without—in the human body and most importantly between man and God.

These medical details are given to prove that there is *forgiveness in the blood* and that *without forgiveness, destruction results*. There is forgiveness both internally and externally for those who may be offenders. As the blood interacts in harmony with cells of the body, so also does the blood of Christ creates harmony between the relations of man and the relations between man and God. Much like within the body, death, destruction, crippling, separation, and pain can result from the lack of spiritual and emotional forgiveness.

> And according to the law almost all things are purged with blood, and without shedding of blood there is no remission. (Heb. 9:22 NKJV)

> For this is my blood of the new covenant, which is shed for many for the remission of sins. (Matt. 26:28)

It is only through the blood that forgiveness can occur because there is forgiveness in the blood. Ultimately, Christ shed His blood once and for all so that we could find forgiveness and harmony with God. As evidenced by the above scriptures, forgiveness is unobtainable without the shedding of blood; more importantly, though, it is not through the blood of infants or animals demanded by a bloodthirsty god. On the contrary, complete and total forgiveness came through a sacrifice of His own—the shed blood of the perfect Lamb of God—Jesus. For no one took His life; He laid it down willingly (John 10:15).

Complete forgiveness could not be accomplished through the blood of rams, bulls, doves, or goats, as they are *foreign to man*, no more than a man could receive a blood transfusion from an animal and live. The blood of animals was merely a *temporizing measure* requiring annual sacrifices to make atonement between man and God. Nevertheless, everlasting forgiveness could only be accomplished by One of *similar likeness or identity* (type specific blood) that could endure the same pain, sufferings, and strive with the worst the world could offer, yet remain blameless and pure. It took the blood of man's Creator to provide the ultimate solution to man's deadliest disease that is sin. The chapter of Isaiah 53 states it so plainly. "And the Lord has laid on Him the iniquity of us all (Isa. 53:6)."

Forgiveness is a must on *three levels*. First and most important, as already discussed, there must be forgiveness between God and man (Please read: 2 Chron. 7:14; Rom. 5:12–21). Second, and at least as important, there must be forgiveness between men as it is impossible to maintain a relationship with God and harbor unforgiveness with your brother, sister, parent, or friend (Matt. 6:12–15; Mark 11:25). Third, which is commonly unrecognized, there must be forgiveness within one's self (Pss. 32; 38:4–10; 69:1–10) as the Psalmist proclaims joy with forgiveness and otherwise torment of the soul. If any of these levels of forgiveness are not attained, the individual will suffer pain, heartache, sickness, self-destruction, and death. The two girls I wrote about earlier had no forgiveness in their bodies as their immune system was set on auto-destruct. The principle is no less apparent in spiritual, psychological, and emotional things.

As there has been a close connection with physical disease, health, and forgiveness throughout the scriptures (Pss. 38; 69; 32; Luke 5:20–23), there must be forgiveness in order for there to be physical, emotional, mental, and spiritual health. I have witnessed countless patients crippled with ailments triggered by mental and emotional bondage initiated by past hurt and emotional injury. Yet, regardless of subjective claims, objective data, or empirical research, there is no amount of expensive medications, chemotherapy, remedies, or antidepressants to substitute the cleansing of the conscience and soul through the shed blood of Christ.

Has someone hurt you beyond your ability to bear? Have you been abused, neglected, or assaulted by a parent, friend, or loved one? Has your trust been broken, causing embarrassment and emotional pain? Is your mind plagued by bitter or angry memories of a past horror? Have you done something so evil that you feel no one could ever forgive? Then, take a moment to pray this prayer and experience the peace, healing, and deliverance that forgiveness can bring as God will bury it in the sea of forgetfulness and cast it as far as the east is from the west. Pray this prayer:

Heavenly Father, I am consumed by the pains in
my past. I am bitter about things that have been
done to me all my life. I am angry with myself
and others over things I cannot control. I hate
the things I have done and am awfully ashamed.
In Jesus's name, I forgive all who have hurt me
because You have forgiven me. I let go of the
bitter past, this very moment, because it is too
great for me to carry any longer. Finally, I ask to
be forgiven for all the things I have done, said,
and failed to do in my life asking that all is covered by Your blood, in Jesus's name.

Make no mistake about it—there is no forgiveness or
healing without the shedding of blood because true, lifesaving
forgiveness is only found in the *blood of Christ*.

FORGIVENESS

On my knees again asking forgiveness,

For a lost, lonely soul such as this.

With no place to hide and nowhere to run,

I come before you, Lord, with my life undone.

A moment of sin, breeding a heart in pain,

As I wait here in hope of your love again.

I cannot find the words in open frustration,

But lift my hands, to grasp Your relation.

For, I cannot live without You, Lord,

Nor can I mend this heart so torn.

Living without Your presence so near,

I cannot breathe in hope, but fear.

Please come into my life once more,

Fill my heart, Lord; I open the door.

Please forgive this sorrow-filled heart,

And restore to him the love only You can impart.

—Ike Pauli MD

Chapter Five

CLEANSING IN THE BLOOD

Once again, I found myself on call, exhausted, hungry, and in desperate need of a shower. Late at night, after being on my feet for nearly twenty hours, I found myself standing in an examining room, staring at a thirteen-year-old girl transferred from northern Wisconsin, who appeared very ill. She was pale, weak, and doubled over in pain. She had been admitted for bloody diarrhea, high blood pressure, and repeated vomiting. Her story was quite classic: she had eaten a "cannibal" sandwich (containing raw hamburger meat) at a tailgate party of a Packer game and a few days later began having severe abdominal cramps, bloody diarrhea, lethargy, fevers, dizziness, and decreased urination. By the time we saw her, she had become severely anemic, had irregular bruising, and had almost no urine output.

This was one sick child, which was confirmed by her laboratory tests that showed severe anemia, low numbers of clotting cells (platelets), and kidney failure. She had the most common cause of renal failure in children: hemolytic uremic syndrome (HUS) associated with a number of infectious illnesses but none more common than the infamous *E. coli 0157 H7* found often in undercooked or raw hamburger meat. The toxin released from the bacteria in the intestines induces a violent response in the body's immune system, indirectly resulting in all the symptoms this young lady was presenting.

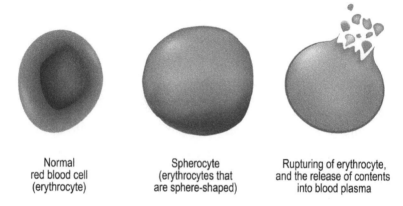

| Normal
red blood cell
(erythrocyte) | Spherocyte
(erythrocytes that
are sphere-shaped) | Rupturing of erythrocyte,
and the release of contents
into blood plasma |

Usually, this disease causes acute-onset vomiting and diarrhea, is self-limited, and if dealt with appropriately, won't need hospitalization. Supportive measures at home such as fluid restriction, bed rest, and blood pressure regulation are all that is needed. Unfortunately, we watched her become more ill with each passing day. Her indicators of kidney function—potassium, phosphates, blood urea nitrogen, creatinine, and acid levels within the blood—became dangerously high, forcing us to place her on renal dialysis. She was in acute renal failure. In other words, her kidneys had failed, allowing multiple waste products from her body's metabolic processes to build up in her blood, and if not removed, she would die.

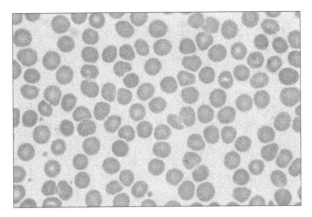

Microscopic view of blood sample with normal red blood cells

The blood is the medium by which the body's nutrients and wastes are exchanged, balanced, neutralized, and transferred. Though her blood was flowing, it was unable to deposit those wastes for elimination. The kidneys, liver, and lungs are the primary sites by which those wastes are eliminated through urine, bile, and respiration. If the wastes and toxins are not eliminated, the body becomes poisoned and quickly dies.

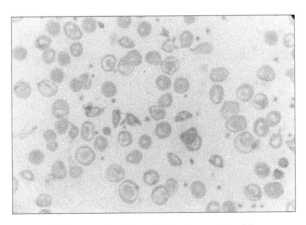

Microscopic view of blood sample with
hemolyzed (destroyed) red blood cells

The blood that Christ shed for man is no different. It flowed from the heart of Christ, through a lost and dying world, removing sin, and depositing it in the sea of forgetfulness (Mic. 7:19). It is only through the blood of Jesus that the toxins, poisons, and wastes our carnal lives continually produce can be removed. This is exactly the process of sanctification: the daily, continuous cleansing the blood of Jesus produces. Unless the blood ceases to flow, with Christ, the sinful wastes are removed continuously. Unlike the blood of animals shed on the Day of Atonement, sins are no longer fleetingly covered and forgiven until the next sacrifice, but cleansed and removed continuously for all who confess and repent (Lev. 16:15–28).

Simply, just because we shower once doesn't mean we shower only once per year, or we never have the need to shower again. Living in a sin-filled world in a carnal body presents challenges to the best of us and may require daily cleansing. Likewise, we don't need to shower a dozen times to remove dirt that has already been washed off. In other words, we daily ask for forgiveness of our transgressions through the blood of Christ, but we need not ask for forgiveness a dozen times a day for the same iniquity because the sin has been eliminated.

Medically, there is no permanent substitute for the functions that the blood performs through the kidneys in removing waste, toxins, and fluid regulation. Using kidney dialysis is only a temporary measure. Such is the difference between forgiveness and the continuous process of sanctification. Forgiveness cures the disease; cleansing clears the debris and removes all traces of illness. Spiritually, there is no substitute for the cleansing power that the blood of Jesus provides (Heb. 9:12–14).

Repression of feelings, suppression of past hurts, rationalization of sin, and denial of sin are all temporizing, poor coping mechanisms for an immature, sin-tattered life. For each person must come to the cross of Christ, face his or her sin, confess it, repent, and ask for the cleansing of His blood to purge his soul. God will then wash him whiter than snow (Ps. 51:7) and remember it no more. "But if we walk in the light as He is in the light, we have fellowship with one another, and the blood of Jesus Christ His Son cleanses us from all sin (1 John 1:7 NKJV)."

It is a simple physical and spiritual principle that without the cleansing blood, death will result from the toxic waste of sin, disease, rebellion, and separation from God.

We were able to dialyze this young girl for nearly nine days until her kidneys began to function again. Dialysis was a temporary replacement for what her body could not do. As a result, she lived despite the threat of her disease. Just as in the Old Testament, the blood of lambs and bulls proved to be a deferring substitute covering the sins of men. There is no alternative, however, for the blood of Jesus. For it is only the blood of Christ Jesus that cleanses us from all unrighteousness. There is no sin so filthy or dirty, no stain so deep, that His blood cannot cleanse. Regardless of what one may have done, the blood provides total cleansing—constantly and forever. If it were not so, Christ would have died in vain.

> To Him who loved us and *washed* us from our
> sins in *His own blood*, and has made us kings
> and priests to His God and Father. (Rev. 1:5–6)

Regardless of the sin, the skeleton in the closet or the goat that has returned from the wilderness (Lev. 16:22), one should never forget there is total cleansing in the blood.

Do you have some secret sin in your life? Do you have some demon from the past that tortures your thoughts and steals your peace? Do you fear the failures of the past as you step into the future? You have heard the old adage that confession is good for the soul but unless you have tried it, you have no idea. If not, take a few moments to tap into the heart of God through Christ and be cleansed by the ever-free-flowing blood of Jesus. You will truly experience then that His perfect love casts out all fear.

> Have mercy upon me, O God, According to Your
> lovingkindness; According to the multitude of
> your tender mercies, *Blot out* my transgres-
> sions. *Wash* me thoroughly from my iniquity
> and *cleanse* me from my sin. For I acknowledge
> my transgressions, and my sin is ever before me.
> Against You, you only, have I sinned, and done
> this evil in Your sight—That You may be found
> just when You speak, And blameless when You
> judge. (Ps. 51:1–4)

THE CRIMSON TIDE

Many bridges have I burned to my distant past,
Yet a horror still lurks, behind a shadow last.
No pattern or reason for what was left behind,
No understanding for the memories, left in my mind.
Though my eyes be fixed on the trail ahead,
And my dreams suspended on a sea of red,
I still feel the anchor of certain memories,
And the pull of a net as I fall on my knees.
The fog of memories remains vivid but can't block my way,
As I am fixed on the Lighthouse to brighten my days.
For as the ashes of a distant past may blow by,
The dust cannot close or cloud my eyes.
And though the skeletons of my past may surface above,
They lose their fear in a sea of blood.
I have learned they have no substance, grip, or blame,
They establish no deed, title, or claim.
They have no power or weapon to wield,
They have no nest or stronghold to build.
It is a wave of blood that has set me free,
Cleansed my life and delivered me.
A most powerful and swift crimson tide,
That forever flows through my new renewed mind.

—Ike Pauli, MD

Chapter Six

HARMONY, PEACE, AND UNITY IN THE BLOOD

BEEP ... BEEP ... BEEP ... I sat straight up in bed. We've all heard the noise, but to a senior resident on call it is a sound that makes your heart lodge in your throat. I jumped out of bed and slipped on my shoes in a single stride, leaped to open the call room door in the black of night, and attempted to read the message on my beeper. I ran to the elevator in full stride when the operator paged overhead, "Code 7 IICU . . . Room 461B . . . Code 7 IICU . . . Room 461B." It seemed as though it took ten minutes to cross the corridors to the room when it was less than sixty seconds. During that minute, a hundred things must have crossed my mind as I tried to replay everything I had learned in the past six years.

I arrived in the room and noticed an army of personnel working hard to save a young girl's life. The anesthesiologist was ventilating her with a bag and mask, the intensive care doctor was calling for epinephrine, another of my colleagues was performing chest compressions, the pharmacist was busily drawing up medications, and a host of nurses were delivering the medications and recording the events. I quickly noted that she was blue (cyanotic) and looked at the monitor and what I noted made my heart skip a beat—ventricular tachycardia.

Immediately, I recognized it as a shockable rhythm and called for the paddles. The intensivist grabbed the paddles and yelled, "200 joules. Clear." As I watched her body lift from the table, "300 joules. Clear." . . . "One milligram of epi . . . 360 joules. Clear." By that time, not only had the patient's heart stopped, but my heart stopped, too. There was no effect. I quickly drew an arterial blood gas and it showed that her oxygen level was extremely low. Since the anesthesiologist was ventilating her with a bag and mask and her chest was moving as breaths were given, we then listened to her breath sounds again, which were strong and equal on both sides.

Things were just not adding up because her oxygen level should have been much higher, and she was not responding to our efforts. By now, her pupils were fixed and dilated, and she had no signs of brain activity. Her heart was fibrillating and then flatlined and we knew we had done everything. "Time of death 01:20 a.m." We had been trying to revive her for thirty minutes and were forced to make the difficult decision to quit. The intensive care doctor had to perform the hardest task of all—telling her parents that their child had died.

During those brief moments, we were perplexed as to why this young lady had died. She had just been placed on a bedpan and, when checked not five minutes later, was discovered to be unconscious. In retrospect, shortly thereafter, it clicked as to what took the life of this precious teen. The answer was contained in her medical history.

At a young age, she was discovered to have a severe congenital heart defect that required several surgical procedures that would not cure her but simply sustain her life until a transplant would eventually be needed. Her heart had finally reached that point of failure and required transplantation. Her perfusion and circulation were so poor, it became obvious what had happened.

With poor circulation, blood tends to pool or sludge in the deep veins, especially those in the legs. Being bedridden, with poor circulation and cardiac problems, all create the right circumstances for a condition called a pulmonary embolus. A pulmonary embolus is simply a large blood clot that travels from the lower extremities, up through the heart, and suddenly blocks blood flow to the lungs. If it is large enough (a saddle embolus), it will cause instant death. There is, unfortunately, no medical intervention to stop it once the clot obstructs the artery.

The body maintains a delicate homeostasis or balance. The heart circulates the blood and with adequate function, does so quite well, responding almost instantaneously to changes in blood pressure, internal and external demands, and position. The muscles also aid in circulation by helping blood return to the heart through movement and exercise. The kidneys filter the blood, adjust blood pressure, and monitor acidity within the blood. The lungs act as an exchange medium between the body and the air, trading carbon dioxide for oxygen, which fuels the body's machinery. It is a complex, metabolic, physiologic relationship, maintaining perfect balance as long as each part of the system is functioning properly.

Stop and think about it for a moment. Every organ is both energized, oxygenated, and fueled by the blood and services the blood (transporting, filtering, detoxing, and oxygenating). Therefore, the blood is the single unifying factor between all of these highly complex processes and organs. Looking at it another way, the blood is the wire between circuits; the fuel and oil for an engine; the coolant for a radiator; the water in a pipe, and much, much more. Ultimately, if the blood does not circulate or serve its function, the body dies.

I remember walking into the pediatric intensive care unit (PICU) to see my first post-operative heart patient of that rotation. My patient was a two-week-old beautiful baby boy who had been diagnosed with a hypoplastic left heart and was only a few days out from his first surgery. As I walked to the side of his bed, the first things that caught my attention were the yellow mesh covering his chest and his total body swelling. As I walked closer I noticed that underneath a clear mesh covering his chest was a beating heart! This was my first experience with an incomplete closure of a postoperative heart repair. I knew that with some of the more complex heart surgeries, there is so much swelling that if the chest was closed, it would squeeze the heart and prevent it from pumping. I also knew that this child had one of the most difficult repairs—the first stage of several very complex surgeries. Yet, I was still not prepared for this incredible sight!

A hypoplastic left heart syndrome is a condition that results when the left side of the heart is underdeveloped, forcing the right side to do the work of both. The condition carries a high mortality due to the complexity of the condition. I have been involved in the care, diagnosis, and transportation of dozens of infants and children with this condition. Their care is very tenuous, their repairs are complex, and their postoperative care seems the most critical. Of all of the heart conditions I have taken care of, the hypoplastic left heart is the most difficult and unpredictable.

As I studied the IVs, I counted eight; all containing some form of critical medication to sustain his life. He had a breathing tube, was on a ventilator delivering very high pressures, had blood pressure monitors, and electrical leads running directly from his heart. His skin was mottled, pale, and with a blue hue. As I studied his chart and his blood work, my heart sank. I counted nearly twenty medications that he was on. His blood work, high ventilator settings, constant requirement for blood products, continuous need for medications to stimulate the heart and increase blood pressure, and overall body swelling gave me a sense of impending doom. I could tell his heart, liver, and kidneys were failing, and that his lungs were filling with fluid. He was experiencing what some would call systemic inflammatory response syndrome (SIRS), a condition similar to adult respiratory distress syndrome, which results in total body shutdown.

Through the weeks that I spent with the family, I realized that the mood had changed from one of hope to one of despair and lack of direction. Our critical care team had done everything, and it didn't seem that anything was changing his course. It seemed like when we plugged one hole in the dam, another opened up worse than the first. We finally reached the decision together—to quit. I will never forget that day. When the ventilator was stopped, the nurse and I pulled the IVs from his swollen little body, and tears filled my eyes. It was then that I set that precious child in his parents' arms for the last time while he took his last few breaths and his last few heartbeats.

Giving them their privacy, I walked to the window that was frosted over. I wiped the fog away and peered out the newly-cleared glass. It was snowing. Regaining my composure, I watched how this fresh, new snow covered the dirty ground. It was beautiful. I wished at that moment that the snow would cover this point in time, the pain and the heartache of this precious baby's parents. I learned that day how powerless I can be as a man and a physician.

I found out that day that there comes a time to stop and to let God's will prevail. In spite of what I had learned, my heart hurt for the family. I couldn't take it anymore. I watched too many children die that month. I went home that night and did something I had never done. I broke down and cried myself to sleep.

The purpose of the heart is to pump or circulate the blood. The blood must be circulated, filtered, oxygenated, and carefully regulated for the body to function properly. If there are defects in any system, it can spell disaster for the whole. As in the infant who had the hypoplastic left heart, the blood could not be circulated in a way needed to sustain life. When the blood cannot be circulated properly, the kidneys, liver, and other organs fail. As in the first young lady, if the blood becomes stagnant, it clots and loses its function.

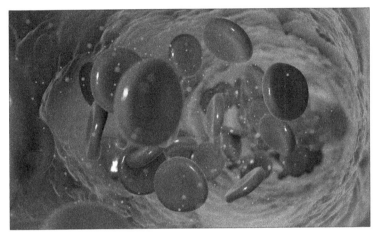

Image of red blood cells flowing through an artery

Such is the blood of Christ as its purpose is to give man unity with God. It is the critical substance that has united a holy God with a sinful man. It is only through the blood of Christ that we have communication, forgiveness, and life. Not only does it give us unity, but it also gives us harmony with God. Ultimately, it was Christ's death and His death alone that ended the enmity between God and man. The blood must flow continuously to accomplish its purpose. The moment the blood of Christ is rejected or neglected to function in the life of a believer, spiritual death results.

Furthermore, the more we rely on "religious" man-made rules and doctrines to define our relationship with God, the more judgmental, self-righteous, and divided we become as believers and the church. These are misplaced and misdirected identities, fracturing the church. The church suffers from it. I often wonder what would happen if all the denominations united under one banner—the blood of Christ.

I remember as a senior resident receiving a call about a three-month-old infant who was being transported from an out-lying hospital for severe croup. Croup is a condition caused by an infection of the windpipe and lower bronchial tree within the lungs that can cause severe swelling that could result in obstruction of the windpipe that rarely results in suffocation. The emergency room had apparently treated him several times with an inhaled medication used to reduce the swelling in the windpipe called racemic epinephrine and intravenous (IV) steroids in an endeavor to shrink the possible swelling of his windpipe with minimal results.

When he reached the floor, however, I could find no evidence of respiratory difficulty or stridor (a high-pitched noise made by a closing windpipe). I couldn't figure it out—this baby was supposed to be sick. Throughout the night, I kept an eye on him and found no signs of a sick child. The following morning, I walked in his room to find a nurse caring for him as he was having "an episode" that looked more to me like a seizure rather than a croup attack. It only lasted sixty seconds, but in that time, we stabilized his airway, giving him supplemental oxygen. I then ordered a battery of tests and labs to work up what apparently was a seizure and not croup. Hours later, I had my answer. The calcium level in his blood was half of what it should have been, and his phosphorous level was twice normal. So what? This infant was not merely having seizures but having bouts of muscle spasms (tetany) so severe that his vocal cords were affected, as well (he quite obviously did not have croup).

There are only a few disorders that can cause this condition, one of which is hypoparathyroidism. It is a big word for when the parathyroid gland fails to secrete or release a hormone to maintain calcium in the blood and body. Furthermore, upon a more complete workup, we found him to have DiGeorge's syndrome. This is a rare condition caused by an abnormality with the twenty-second chromosome leading to heart defects, low calcium due to underdeveloped or absent parathyroid glands, and defects in the immune system.

By determining the nature of his illness, we were hopefully able to appropriately treat him. By giving him the right hormones and calcium, we treated his calcium problem. His heart anomaly was unremarkable or insignificant and would not need treatment. We would not be able to correct his immune defect though. This would be a long battle throughout his whole life. What's the point? *A simple defect on a single chromosome affected the whole body in several different ways through the blood.* One part of the defect of the chromosome affects the blood's metabolism, one affects the blood via the immune system, and the other affects the flow of blood. One defect affects the whole.

The Book of Romans (Rom. 12:4–5) tells us that we are of one body in Christ. Each of us are members of the same body. We are not only united to God through Christ's blood but also one another. Truly the blood is also the unifying factor in the body of Christ. It is only the blood of Jesus that gives us the opportunity to be connected as one body. It is only through the work of the Holy Spirit that harmony can be maintained. As in the infant above who had a defect in chromosome twenty-two that affected his entire body, the body of Christ would be non-existent and become dysfunctional without the shed blood of Jesus uniting us as believers.

Driving my point home, 1 Corinthians 10:16 (KJV) tells us, "The cup of blessing which we bless, is it not the *communion* of the blood of Christ?" Even the Latin root word from which we get the term *communion* is the same origin of the words common, unity, and community.[1] Thus, it was even under-stood centuries ago that the symbol of partaking the blood of Christ during the partaking of communion was a unifying factor within the body of Christ.

Without the blood, we have no circulation, no communica-tion, and no unity. In another light, for years and across many cultures, man has exchanged his blood with someone close as a "blood brother" to symbolize a committed, inseparable relation-ship between those who are unrelated. This action symbolized a union or brotherhood that in many ways went beyond even the strongest family ties. Likewise, Jesus's blood has made us as believers in Christ "blood brothers," adopting us into a united family, one body, to His glory and our benefit. Like it or not, no matter the "denomination," if you are a believer in Christ, pur-chased by His blood, then you are a part of the body of Christ, unified with Him and with one another.

At that time you were without Christ, being aliens from the commonwealth of Israel and strangers from the covenants of promise, having no hope and without God in the world. But now in Christ Jesus you who once were far off have been made *near* by the *blood* of Christ. For He Himself is our peace, who has made both *one*, and has *broken down* the middle *wall of division* between us, having abolished in His flesh the enmity, that is, the law of commandments contained in ordinances, so as to create in Himself *one new man* from the two, thus making peace, and that He might reconcile them both to God in **one** body through the cross, thereby putting to death the enmity. And He came and preached peace to you who were near. For through Him we both have access by *one Spirit* to the Father. Now, therefore, you are no longer strangers and foreigners, but fellow *citizens* with the saints and *members of the household* of God, having been built on the foundation of the apostles and prophets, Jesus Christ Himself being the chief cornerstone, in whom the whole building, being joined together, grows into a holy temple in the Lord, in whom you also are being built together for a habitation of God in the Spirit. (Eph. 2:11–22 NKJV)

I was an only child to my parents. When I returned to the church at fifteen years of age, my mother was living in Chicago, and my father told me that if I wanted to start going to church, I was going to have to find my own way. So, leaders in our youth group and my uncle, who also recently received Christ, would switch off taking me to and from church for months until my grandmother bought me a car. This once-lonely, latch-key, only child found himself in the midst of a new family—a family of a different kind.

My Cornerstone church family through youth ministry, home ministries, and even my pastor's family began to adopt me into their lives, homes, and activities. I was no longer alone, isolated, and rejected but a part of a new family that really loved and cared about me—for who I was. I found joy and began to laugh. They accepted this nerdy, quirky, and ostracized teen who had nothing to offer without condition.

Even today, I still have many of these relationships for nearly forty years within my Cornerstone family. I met my wonderful wife of over thirty-five years at church, married at my church, was instructed at my church, and was discipled at my church. My Cornerstone family has given me love, encouragement, a platform, and a medium to use my talents to serve Christ. I have often said, "Jesus saved my soul—but my church saved my life." That is a personal testimony of the power of love and unity established by the blood of Christ through the church.

The first two young lives described earlier tragically died prematurely because the mechanisms for the flow of blood were defective. They had severe congenital heart defects that did not allow the blood to perform its function and communicate with the rest of the body. Without that communication, the natural harmony within their bodies could not be maintained. The third, however, we were able to treat, hopefully adding years to his life. The blood of Jesus is the communication and harmony in the believer's life. So, it is important that the spiritual hearts of men continue to beat with the blood of Christ. Unforgiveness, resentment, bitterness, hate, bigotry, and anti-Semitism are all cancers to the spiritual heart of man and will lead to death. Without the blood of Christ, there is an impenetrable wall between God and man. Thank God, there are harmony and unity in the blood.

Are you searching for a fulfilling relationship? Have your friends, relatives, spouse, and acquaintances hurt you, lied about you, or left you for dead? There can only be one true relationship lived without pain or fear of abandonment or rejection. That relationship is with your heavenly Father. He will never leave, abandon, or forsake you. Only He can repair the broken elements in your relationships. For anything to heal, blood must actively flow to the injury; otherwise, it will become infected, develop gangrene, wither, and die. Thus, your life and your relationships can only be kept alive and healed through the ever-flowing blood of Christ. There is *unity in the blood.*

As an act of your will, give up the stubbornness of heart, forgive anyone who has hurt you, and pray this prayer:

71

Please, God, forgive me of my sins, bitterness, failures, resentment, and hatred. Let your blood flow through me so that I may have unity, harmony, and complete and total restoration into the body of Christ. Don't allow my past hurts to control my future relationships. Don't allow my fears of rejection and pain keep me from loving, enduring, and fruitful relationships in my home, church, and ministry.

PEACE OF MY MIND

In my past pounds a heartless beating,

Where emotions run wild with an intense heating.

As I stand alone wanting to open the door,

I am gripped by confusion, bound to the floor.

I reach out my hand to stable my way,

Trudging through my emotions once again,

While trying to grasp the Truth of life,

Yet the fear too great . . . to pay the price.

I stand so still, twirling inside,

Looking for someplace to run and hide.

While my emotions twist and tumble all about,

They have emptied my mind and filled it with doubt.

I desperately reach for the distant door ahead,

But stammer in the mire of my own dread.

To have peace inside and a moment to share,

That would dim the torment's evil glare.

continued

Standing so calm, yet raging inside,

As hope, word, and faith are there to confide.

Gripping my faith, trying to step outside,

While the chains of my past still shackle my mind.

Now once I drop upon my knees,

And truly trust You with my every need.

I can open the door to my tormented soul,

Allowing Your love, Oh Lord, to fill the hole.

To stand in Your peace is all I ask.

To live my faith, my truest task.

To let your blood cleanse this wayward mind,

Freeing it to soar, once again, as an eagle in flight.

—Ike Pauli MD

Chapter Seven

HEALING IN THE BLOOD

I was working in one of the busiest children's emergency rooms in the country, late at night. Well over fifty-thousand visits per year have poured through that emergency room at upwards of over one hundred-thirty patients per day. It was one of those days when we were already ten to fifteen patients behind, and the night had just started. It was noisy, controlled chaos, as doctors and nurses were running all over the emergency room trying to keep up with the barrage of sick children pouring through the door. Worse yet, we had just had two traumas flown in via helicopter. I was rushing to see my next patient when I heard, "Dr. Pauli, we need you in room two . . . Now!" I ran into the room and found a three-year-old boy unresponsive and very pale. He was sweating profusely, had spontaneous respirations, a rapid heart rate, and obviously poor perfusion.

As I completed my secondary survey, I found out that earlier this week he had been seen at an outlying emergency room for an inner-lip laceration. Apparently, it was severe enough that the doctors thought it required stitches. The parents, however, noticed that throughout the week he had been vomiting blood and passing thick, black stools. They had taken him back to the same emergency room several times, but they would do nothing, though his lip continued to bleed excessively. I quickly placed an IV, drew blood for lab work, and typed and cross-matched him. We then infused him with fluids and ordered, "O negative blood STAT."

Blood group

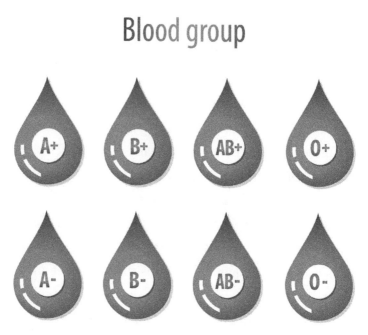

Different blood groups in humans

I started to get a little nervous as I probed the inner aspect of his lip laceration and noted an arterial bleeder pulsating blood into his mouth. I called for my attending as I applied pressure to the wound. He quickly arrived, and we re-sutured the wound after closing and tying off the arterial bleeder. By this time, the child had regained consciousness and was fighting us like a normal three-year-old. After he was stabilized, and the O negative blood was running in his veins, the results of his lab work began to return. I couldn't believe my eyes; his hematocrit (a measure of his red blood cells) was 12 percent (the normal range was 32–35 percent). He had actually lost nearly two-thirds of his blood volume. Because of this, I slowed the blood infusion rate down and decided to give him less volume as too much blood infused in a severely anemic person can throw them into heart failure. We admitted him to the intensive care unit that night for further observation and treatment.

The next morning, as I thought about this small boy and his big problem, I realized that the arterial bleeder in his lip was not the whole answer to the bleeding that this child experienced. Labs drawn the following morning helped to confirm my suspicion. This child had a clotting disorder called factor nine deficiency or hemophilia B. His condition was previously undetected and masked until he had a deep cut, which proved to be life-threatening.

It was another day in the same hospital, now making rounds on the general medicine ward, and I remember walking the floors in the early morning hours, making my usual rounds when I heard the code bell sound. I looked over my shoulder, and my heart skipped a beat as a nurse screamed for my assistance echoing across the floor. I ran into the room and found a little twelve-month-old boy unconscious with blood pouring out of his nose and mouth. The nurse was so stunned that I had to yell to get her attention, "Get me the bag and mask now!" I then began to give him artificial respirations and ordered the placement of an oral gastric tube. As we attempted to place the tube, he vomited an incredible amount of blood, so much that it covered his entire abdomen and nearly hit me in the face two feet away. I then called for "two units of platelets, DDAVP, and O negative blood—STAT!" We paged the ENT, and by that time the intensive care staff arrived to assist.

Knowing his history, I knew that the most likely source of bleeding was in his nose. So, I placed phenylephrine in his nose, hoping to slow the bleeding. The decision was then made to better control his airway, so I managed to place a breathing tube in him beneath the pools of blood within his nose, mouth, and windpipe. As I secured his airway, the ENT specialist then packed his nose to control the remaining hemorrhage. We then rushed him to the PICU for stabilization and further treatment.

This child had a rather devastating series of events that led up to this moment. At a few months of age, his intestines had twisted due to a congenital deformity, which caused his gut to be strangulated and die. Consequently, nearly all of his small intestines had to be surgically removed. And because he had no intestines, he required intravenous nutrition. Now, the prolonged intravenous nutrition resulted in liver disease and possible liver failure.

Liver failure creates a whole cascade of new problems, one of which is a failure in the production of clotting factors. If there are no clotting factors, there is bleeding and an impaired ability for the body to repair itself. This child had reached that point. He had been chronically hospitalized because of bleeding and recurrent infections. This allowed him to be well-known among nurses and hospital staff.

Until now, his bleeding problems had been quite routine. If he began to bleed, pressure would be applied to his nose with an ice pack for ten minutes. If that didn't work, he would be infused with a medicine known to help clotting, and if that failed, then he would be infused with blood products to replace the low clotting factors. Though this regimen became quite routine, I warned my interns that his condition could be quite serious if he really began to bleed for I had experienced this before. He bled this time during the direct pressure stage, enough to cause him to lose consciousness and nearly die, something no one really seemed to be prepared for. Though initially stabilized, his condition worsened over the next week as a result of his devastating blood loss and inability to heal. He later died of fatal hemorrhage and systemic inflammatory response while on a ventilator in the intensive care unit.

There are remarkably well-balanced and regulated chains of events in the blood that occur with tissue injury within the body. The chains of events are so complex and detailed that they exceed the scope of this book. Modern medicine has only recently put all of the pieces together. Nevertheless, simply stated, damaged tissues release proteins, which attract clotting cells called platelets. These platelets in turn release proteins that promote further accumulation of platelets, activation of enzymes, and activation of protein bridges that form a temporary barrier until the tissues heal. With the barrier in place, the immune system regulates further repair and guards against infection through highly complex and specific chemical interactions between the body's blood vessels and immune system.

It sounds complex and it is. Most physicians have difficulty understanding the intricacies of clotting and healing. Simply, the blood contains the essential nutrients, vitamins, proteins, and cells to promote healing. If there was no blood, or if the substances and interactions within the blood became faulty, there would be no healing—and death would result. Despite the level of understanding of complex mechanisms within the body, the fact remains that without the blood, there would be no healing. Without healing, life-giving substances bleed away, infection sets in, and death results.

The two children I described above had several things in common. Initially, they had a lack of critical factors in their blood, which prevented them from clotting and triggered near-fatal bleeding. As a result, they bled so excessively that their bodies could not compensate without intervention, producing near death in one and, tragically, death in another. Finally, their conditions were chronic, having no cure, and having profound effects on the remainder of their lives. It is true then, that there is healing within the blood and without the blood there is death.

In that light, the concept doesn't seem so profound when we read that there is healing through the blood of Christ—for our bodies, minds, souls, and spirits. Isaiah describes it perfectly:

> Surely He has borne our griefs and carried our
> sorrows: yet we esteemed Him stricken, smitten
> by God, and afflicted. But he was wounded for

our transgression, He was bruised for our iniq-
uities; the chastisement for our peace was upon
Him, and by his stripes we are healed. (Isa.
53:4–5 NKJV)

By understanding that the blood is the source of the body's
healing, one can more fully understand that Christ's blood is
the source of healing for the believer's body, soul, and relationships. His blood is supernatural blood not bound, however,
by physical principles and complex interactions, but by incon-
ceivable spiritual truths.

As the two children required life-sustaining transfusions to
support their lives, so also Christ has provided a single life-sustaining transfusion for those who choose to believe. I find it
quite ironic that even though He had ascended to the Father and
returned perfected, Jesus still had his wounds. His flesh had no
blood, though. He gave it all at Calvary—for a sick, injured,
and dying world. His wounds remind us that He bore our sickness and disease. I also find it amazing that a substance (the
blood) once forbidden to drink, now becomes the sole source
of life, health, and forgiveness. We are commanded to partake
that substance in His remembrance:

Most assuredly, I say to you, unless you eat the
flesh of the Son of Man and drink His blood,
you have no life in you. Whoever eats My flesh
and drinks My blood has eternal life, and I will
raise him up at the last day. For My flesh is

food indeed, and My blood is drink indeed.
(John 6:54–56)

Yes, it is the uncorrupted blood of Jesus shed once and for all
to deliver, heal, save, and restore. Such lends to the importance
of the communion and the penalty for partaking unworthily.
For if death and illness result from an unworthy communion,
how much more are there life and healing through that taken
(worthily) in faith, hope, remembrance, and forgiveness (1 Cor.
11:27–30). It is no wonder the church is commissioned to partake of this communion often in remembrance of Christ. Take
communion often: Take it at church, take it as a family, take it
as a Bible study, and take it worthily. As my pastor says, "It is
the meal that heals." So, it must be always remembered when
Matthew 26:26–29 is read and the Holy Communion is par-
taken: there is complete and total *healing in the blood.*

Do you face a debilitating disease or some crippling dis-
ability? Diseases like lupus, rheumatoid arthritis, Cancer,
AIDS, schizophrenia, Lyme's, and leukemia all strike fear into
the hearts of men and women. Our God, however, has made
a provision for healing his children where there needs to be
no fear. Is your heart broken and trampled beneath the feet of
a cold, cruel world? Well, God has made a provision for you,
too! I can assure you that there is no wound too deep, wide, or
severely infected that the blood of Jesus cannot heal. The only
thing preventing your healing is ignorance and interruption in
blood flow (not asking or a lack of faith).

This very moment, this very hour, call upon the name of the Lord and ask for the healing power of the Holy Spirit through the blood of Christ to heal any and all of your infirmities. "Father, right now I forgive all of those who have hurt or conspired against me. Now, allow the blood that was shed on the cross for my healing to flow through my veins, initiating and completing the healing within my body, my mind, and in my spirit, in Jesus's name."

LONELY ROAD

On a cobblestone road walks the shadow of a man,

Bearing a load no one else could stand.

Trudging on in anguish, each step in pain,

While His accusers crowd around and curse His name.

Driven on his path being beaten in anger,

By those notorious for pointing their fingers,

At something . . . no one really knows,

For something . . . He is taking these awesome blows.

As his flesh becomes torn and beaten,

He reaches the Skull, tattered and weakened.

Pound by pound being nailed to a cross,

Between two thieves, only one being lost.

Stripe by stripe, blood flows from his corpse,

Signing the battle has only begun his course,

For as they stand and curse His name,

He lays down his life for their own gain.

Yet, the battle is not over when they seal the tomb,

And peer upon him with eternal gloom.

For, when they see that stone rolled away,

They then will know that He rose from the grave.

—Ike Pauli MD

Chapter Eight

PROTECTION IN THE BLOOD

Trial by fire seems to be the theme of my medical career. I have rarely been afforded the luxury of easing into something. My peers and subordinates began to hate the times when I was on call because they knew some catastrophe would likely unfold. In medicine, we call it a "black cloud." While my days and call nights haven't necessarily been episodes of *ER* or *Code Black*, they could probably come close. Because of this background, even to this day, I take call with great apprehension, wondering what could possibly happen next. However, I wouldn't trade my experiences for anything. Each experience has afforded me invaluable knowledge, insight, personal growth, and helped me become the physician I am.

It was my first week on service in the pediatric intensive care unit as a third-year medical student. This rotation taught me more about the blood than any other. As usual, while I was still learning the ropes of a new rotation, a six-month-old baby boy was admitted to my care. I had never seen anything like it, and I hope I never will again. Once again, I was not prepared for what I was about to experience. I have never seen an infant this sick in my career. He was grunting, ribs were retracting, his nostrils flaring, and was struggling for each breath as if it was his last. Even for a medical student, it wasn't very hard to see that this child was in severe respiratory distress. As I listened to his lungs, I thought they sounded like a wet sponge that was being pressed upon a countertop.

Even as a third-year medical student I realized that this baby was about to die. He was on ten liters of oxygen per minute with a non-rebreather mask delivering 100 percent oxygen to his failing lungs. His eyes were an open book to his deteriorating condition. I will never forget his look of horror, similar to that of someone drowning and reaching out for their last hope, or someone falling off a one-hundred-foot cliff grasping for something to hold. This look will strike fear into any pediatrician—one that I dread seeing even today. I watched his wide-open eyes reaching out in desperation, crying out for me to save his life.

Later that morning, it was clear that he was in full respiratory failure despite everything we had done. We had to intubate him and place him on a mechanical ventilator. This temporarily stabilized him, allowing us to gain a more thorough secondary survey (physical exam). He was a dirty child who had a notably putrid odor of not having been bathed for quite some time. His mouth was full of a cottage cheese-like substance that we later identified as thrush. There was so much it had to physically be removed with a tongue blade. He was also wasted, malnourished, and dehydrated—so much so that I could easily feel his enlarged liver and spleen upon examining his abdomen. I couldn't believe it; he was only one pound over birth weight.

Assuming the worst, we sent a battery of tests to the lab, only to confirm what we already knew. Actually, the infant's social history gave us our diagnosis. He had five other siblings, each by a different father. His mother had also been involved in illicit drug use including heroin, cocaine, and marijuana. There were too many risk factors in a child with such a severe illness and at the top of our list was AIDS.

We started broad-spectrum antibiotics, intravenous nutrition, and attempted to clean the baby up. Throughout the week, things went from bad to worse. We needed to know for sure if it was AIDS, but the diagnosis at that time could be difficult in a six-month-old. The battery of tests trickled in, and they all confirmed our suspicions of the presence of HIV. This precious infant had AIDS. The silver stain resulting from an open lung biopsy confirmed the source of his failing lungs— Pneumocystis carinii pneumonia. There was no doubt about it. Yet, despite knowing his infirmity, being on broad-spectrum antibiotics, and having the best medical care available, we could not save his life.

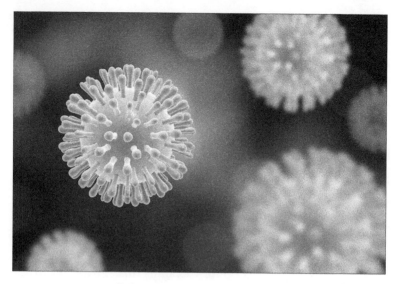

C.G. representation of HIV virus

What is this dreaded disease called AIDS? You may not know what it means to be HIV positive. His mother didn't, even though it has occupied the forefront of advertisements, commercials, and news broadcasts for the last two decades. Before 1985, few knew anything about the illness. Today, it seems that everyone knows something about AIDS. Yet, in spite of her ignorance, she was the one who transmitted the virus to her son. What is it that makes this virus so deadly? Quite simply, the virus is like a stealth bomber. This virus invades the body undetected, grows, multiplies, and destroys the key cells that regulate the body's immune system before adequate defenses can be mounted. What makes it even more lethal is that the virus can remain hidden or dormant for many years until its full manifestation. Even though it may be dormant, it is still equipped to infect another host. The virus manifests itself by destroying the primary regulatory cell of the immune system and as a result, causes AIDS—acquired immunodeficiency syndrome.

HIV Entry to T Cell

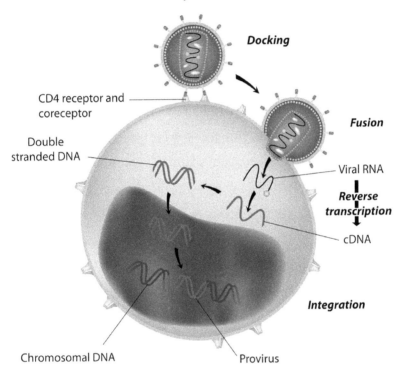

So, what is the point? There is protection in the blood. Without a properly functioning immune system, parasites, bacteria, other viruses, and fungi are able to invade and destroy the body unchecked. With a normally functioning immune system, most of these invaders will cause little more than a fever, runny nose and cough in the normal individual. The vast majority of people with AIDS die from otherwise nonlethal infections and not from the HIV virus itself. With a poorly functioning immune system, any infection can be life-threatening. We need the blood with its immune system intact in order to survive. It is a very dynamic substance — learning day by day, recognizing new invaders, and destroying them at will.

The white blood cells culminate the protective barrier from infection. Just like there are different kinds of soldiers within an army that perform different functions, there are different cells that perform different functions. Neutrophils protect from bacterial infections. Lymphocytes protect against viral invasion. Eosinophils and basophils help regulate allergic reactions, clotting, and help protect in parasitic infections. Monocytes and macrophages consume invaders and present them to the lymphocytes for antibody production. This is extremely oversimplified but suffices to say that the blood is completely dedicated to the protection of its body! All in all, the blood is the first and last defense against any potential assailant or aggressor.

The elements of blood

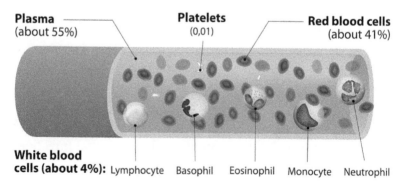

Plasma (about 55%)　　Platelets (0,01)　　Red blood cells (about 41%)

White blood cells (about 4%): Lymphocyte　Basophil　Eosinophil　Monocyte　Neutrophil

I think by now you can see there is a trend. It is the blood of Christ that fights for our protection on a daily basis. It's that first and last piece of armor that sustains our lives. And, it must remain dynamic, constantly utilized by the believer. Each and every day it must be applied to the doorpost of the believer's soul, mind, and body. Protection from what one might ask? Death, the enemy, sickness, disease, and judgment.

> For I will pass through the land of Egypt on that night and will strike all the firstborn in the land of Egypt, both man and beast; and against all the gods of Egypt I will execute judgment: I am the Lord. Now the blood shall be sign for you on the houses where you are. And when I see the blood, I will pass Over you; and the plague shall not be on you to destroy you when I strike the land of Egypt . . . For the Lord will pass through to strike the Egyptians; and when He sees the blood on the lintel and on the two door posts, the Lord will pass over the door posts, the Lord will pass over the door and not allow the Destroyer to come into you houses to strike you And you will observe this thing as an ordinance for you and your sons forever. (Ex. 12:12–13, 23–24 NKJV)

The blood is the crimson shield that permanently identifies us as God's children and recipients of His everlasting covenant.

God's Word is true and His covenants unbreakable. The blood of Christ is that everlasting sign and weapon to all that His children cannot and will not be destroyed by any force or foe.

I have heard many Christians laugh at their enemy and call him defeated. They state that he is an old, toothless, roaring lion without power. Though he may be a defeated foe, he is far from being toothless. Let me paint a picture of this toothless lion. First, the enemy is intelligent. He knows his opponent's weaknesses from a lifetime of observation and patterns of behavior (Rev. 12:10). Second, the enemy is highly organized (Dan. 9:10–14), with the specific purpose (Eph. 6:12), and the ultimate goal to destroy everything created by God (John 10:10). And finally, the enemy is invisible to the naked eye and has specific powers that are beyond our physical vision and understanding, a formidable enemy that apparently has every advantage.

He is a far cry from a toothless lion. Think about it; the believer's enemy knows if he is fearful, worried, or anxious. He knows this because he can see the dilatation of his opponent's pupils, the sweat on his palms and forehead, and the increase in his heart rate and respiratory rate (an enemy that cannot be fooled). He and his legions are ever-present spies, listening to your worries, concerns, fears, and prayers. He can also manipulate physical and spiritual forces against his opponent as he assesses his opponent's vulnerability with focused efforts. Actually, the believer's enemy (the devil) is like the HIV virus, penetrating its host in a moment of weakness or sin and destroying the very fabric of his soul and spiritual defenses through manipulation, intimidation, and domination. Similarly, he may lay in wait and slowly multiply until the opportune moment for destruction.

Thus, the believer's enemy has motive, method, and power to accomplish his goals. Truly, on his own the believer, much less the sinner, does not stand a chance (Heb. 2:14–15). It has been said, however, that "No weapon formed against you shall prosper (Isa. 54:17)." To stand his ground, God Himself has provided through his Son and Spirit an impenetrable fortress to attack, a commission, and armor as described in Ephesians 6:13–18.

The blood is also a vital piece of that armor that provides constant, unending, and impenetrable protection. Have no fear, my fellow believer, *"when the enemy comes in like a flood, the spirit of the Lord will lift up a standard against him* (Isa. 59:19)." The blood of Jesus Christ is that standard.

"And they overcame him by the blood of the Lamb and by the word of their testimony, and they did not love their lives to the death (Rev. 12:11)." There is no doubt or supposition in that scripture. There is not an "if" or "maybe" within those words. So, the believer need not live in fear or doubt, but in confidence and victory. For, no matter the disease, affliction, or weapon, the blood of Christ offers permanent protection as long as it covers the doorposts of his soul. Satan once again becomes a defeated foe *only through the blood of Jesus*. It is a fact then; an undeniable truth in both the physical and spiritual realm. There is protection in the blood.

Do you lie awake at night unable to sleep, occupied and encumbered by the worries of this world? Are you unreasonably afraid of others or fearful to leave your home? Are you bound by phobias (irrational fears) that embarrass and humiliate you? Are you controlled by addictive habits? Live in the confidence that Jesus Christ is Lord and that His blood will cover you, deliver you, and give you protection from all the evils around you.

Know this, as the blood of Christ covers your soul, God Himself shows up to protect and care for you as His very own. As such, there is no adversary, enemy, or destroyer so great that can overcome our God. Have the assurance that nothing in life can overcome or destroy your soul through the blood of Christ.

Lord, I believe and trust You; please let the blood of your Son, that was shed on the cross, cover the doorposts of my soul: that I might have the impenetrable protection of my God. From this moment on, I will overcome by the blood of the Lamb and the word of my testimony. (Rev. 12:11)

Fear not, for I have redeemed you; I have called you by your name; you are mine. When you pass through the waters, I will be with you; And through the rivers, they shall not overflow you. When you walk through the fire, you shall not be burned, nor shall the flame scorch you. (Isa. 43:1–2)

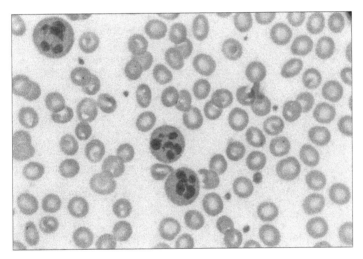

Microscopic view of blood with neutrophils and red blood cells

Chapter Nine

POWER IN THE BLOOD

Would you be free from the burden of sin? There's pow'r in the blood, pow'r in the blood . . . Would you o'er evil a victory win? There's wonderful pow'r in the blood. There's pow'r, pow'r, wonder working pow'r in the blood of the Lamb: There is pow'r pow'r, wonder working pow'r in the precious blood of the Lamb.[2]

It was my final year in residency, and I thought I had experienced it all. At this point in my career, I was ready to be done and go out into the world and practice all that I had learned. This night proved that I still had much to learn. This month I was in the NICU, and once again, tonight I was on call. The other residents, fellow attending physicians, and I had just completed evening rounds when I was informed by the obstetrician on call that a nineteen-year-old girl had been found unconscious on her kitchen floor and that she was twenty-eight weeks pregnant. They wanted us to be on alert because they were unsure of the reason she was unconscious and were concerned that they may have to deliver her emergently while searching for the cause. Their current impression was that she had a ruptured brain aneurysm.

She was home alone, however, and was found unconscious, so no one knew for sure what happened. Did she hit her head, have an overdose, a seizure, or a stroke? In any event, they wanted us on standby because they knew they might have to deliver the premature baby quickly, and they wanted us to be ready. There were no answers, only questions.

Not five minutes later, the phone rang with the message, "Come STAT to Labor and Delivery, number three!" We ran over as fast as we could while pulling the crash cart and transport Isolette. As I ran into the room, I couldn't believe my eyes! Amidst the flurry of activities and noise, my eyes fixed on a limp, blue, lifeless twenty-eight-week-old premature baby lying near-breathless on a cold, stainless steel table. The baby's mother turned for the worst and needed an immediate C-section, or the baby would die. The warmers were still cold, which were critical to raising her body temperature; the resuscitation equipment to help her breathe was still in the cabinets; and she was making minimal effort to breathe on her own.

My first thought was, "How long has that baby been on the table?" My second thought was, "Now this is what I was trained for!" The nurse practitioner began rescue breaths as I prepared the oxygen and intubation equipment. I called for a heart rate and was told that it was sixty beats per minute, so I ordered chest compressions STAT! I then quickly intubated her as the nurse told me that the baby's temperature was ninety-five degrees. Knowing that the infant was critically ill, and having limited equipment, I immediately called for a warming blanket and decided to rush her to the NICU. On the way, we rushed through the halls and the elevators as we continued CPR en route. Once there, we placed her on a ventilator, gave epinephrine to maintain heart rate and blood pressure, IV fluids, and chest compressions.

This obviously wasn't working, so I ordered several more doses of epinephrine to be given and to start a dopamine drip to help maintain renal blood flow and blood pressure. Several doses were given when I called for her temperature. "Ninety-four degrees," was the reply. I knew that we needed to warm her up because the medications we were using were not as effective in hypothermic conditions. It seemed like forever before we were able to increase her temperature. Her sugar level now was 15 mg/dl (normal is greater than 40 mg/dl for a newborn), and her heart rate was still less than one hundred beats per minute. We infused a total of five rounds of epinephrine, bicarbonate, glucose, blood, and finally, after forty-five minutes, we stabilized her.

During this time, some of the nurses were asking me in a whisper, "How far are we going to take this?" I did not feel a release, however, and all the while I was praying for the infant and hoping that what we were doing for her was the right thing. I even looked at my attending on several occasions, searching for a sign of what we could possibly do next. She agreed with each decision, giving us the benefit of her vast experience. We discussed the slim chances this baby girl would have and still decided to press on. The next several hours would tell the tale. Once stable, we would have to give her surfactant to help her premature lungs. Next, we would need to closely follow her electrolytes, nutrition, heart, and kidney function. Would this precious baby have lung, heart, kidney, or brain damage? Did we go too far trying to save her life?

As the evening's events wound down, with the umbilical lines secured, the ventilator set, and the infant's blood pressure stabilized, I was relieved to rest for a few hours. I had now been on my feet for over twenty hours and the only thing that was keeping me going was the adrenaline surge of the evening. I remember lying my head down on the stiff hospital pillow and mattress at nearly 3:00 a.m. and praying for two hours of sleep before another full day started. I began thinking about our evening, staring into the black.

By restoring the flow of blood and oxygen to the tissues in her body, we were able to restore a delicately balanced harmony for circulation, breathing, and nutrients. This premature infant was unable to make this balance on her own at such a young gestational age. We were able to stabilize her and give her the proper nutrition and vitamins her body would require until she was able to feed on her own. We did all of this through the blood. I was quite amazed that over the next several weeks as she made remarkable progress, and by God's grace, had no adverse or long-term complications or problems due to her prematurity. Sadly enough, we were informed her mother, who was found unconscious, died days later of what was determined to be a ruptured brain aneurysm. In spite of this tragedy, however, after spending several weeks in the NICU, I found some comfort, watching her grandmother carry her home—healthy.

She was named after her mother. There is a remarkable source of power and energy in the blood.

On another occasion, I had worked twenty hours straight in the PICU. My feet were aching, my body felt tired, but my mind was racing. Though I thought I was prepared for the day, I didn't know what might happen next as a new day started. Then at 4:00 a.m. we were sent to see a two-year-old Asian boy from the emergency room. This toddler had been vomiting with diarrhea for nearly two days and had become unconscious. When arriving in the emergency room, he was having seizures and had a blood glucose of 10 mg/dl (greater than 60 mg/dl is normal for this age). He was given glucose, intubated, and placed on a ventilator. On further evaluation and discussion during rounds we realized that in spite of having a low blood sugar, he had no ketones in his urine (byproducts produced during fasting states from the breakdown of fats in the body, which are released in the urine). This information helped us narrow down the possibilities of what happened to this child drastically.

Nonketotic hypoglycemia is extremely rare and we knew just who to call — our famous metabolic geneticist. He helped us order the specific tests and diagnose the cause for his coma and seizures. We determined that our patient and children like him are missing a single enzyme that prevents them from breaking down fats. When the body's sugar is burned up, they have no fuel for their body's machinery. In the past, children with this and similar disorders quite frequently died of unknown causes. What is so scary is that these children usually have no symptoms until they get their first bout of vomiting and diarrhea, and they have no way of eating to maintain their blood sugar. As a result, without urgent medical intervention, they may seize, lose consciousness, go into a coma, and die.

This baby was fortunate, however, in that we made the diagnosis in hours. Remarkably, after only a week in the PICU and several weeks in the hospital, he woke up from his coma and went home. I saw him a year later in the hospital, and he was a happy boy. His only lasting effects from the profound and prolonged low blood sugar were a seizure disorder and transient developmental delays. He was, after all, the only son of a large family and thus was even more cherished after a brush with death.

The blood carries the needed fuel for the body's metabolic machinery, which carries thousands of enzymes and hormones that regulate the body's functions. It is the blood that carries proteins, fats, sugars, and oxygen (a fuel) to the tissues and removes carbon dioxide and waste products simultaneously. There is incredible power in the blood. As demonstrated by this two-year-old boy, it is the only factor that contains all of the body's nutrients, vitamins, minerals, oxygen, hormones, sugars, and wastes. The instant the blood stops flowing, the body's machinery slows and then stops, and organ and tissue damage occur in minutes. If a physician needs to know how a patient's liver, heart, and kidneys are functioning, he checks their blood. If he needs to know the patient's nutritional status or lipid profile (cholesterol screening), he checks the blood.

The blood is transportation, temporary storage, and communication for the body's machinery. Without its functions, it would be like trying to run a car or jet without fuel. It would be like trying to turn on a light, appliance, or television without electricity. That is not a profound revelation, just simple physical principles. Things don't run without power or energy: The body is no different as evidenced by this two-year-old with low blood sugar. Even the simplest forms of interactions are governed by the basic laws of matter and energy. For the body, the blood is the sole means of transportation of fuel, power, nutrition, waste transport, and removal. Countless chemical reactions take place each minute within the body, and all are dependent on the blood. So many occur at a given second to maintain a delicate balance of life and consciousness that it is overwhelming even for the brightest medical mind.

I remember being on call as an intern in the intermediate intensive care unit, conducting my rounds on the patients in the unit. It was early in the evening, and everyone was pretty much settled in for the night. The only thing that could be heard was the intermittent beeping of various monitors and a few pulsating ventilators. The next thing I hear is nurses rushing by with my attending wheeling a three-year-old African-American boy on a stretcher.

I walked into the room to assess the status of my new admission. He was on a considerable amount of oxygen, and the nurse told me that he had sickle cell disease and was experiencing acute chest syndrome. As I had seen it a few times before, I knew acute chest syndrome was a serious condition in patients with sickle cell disease that can occur when the blood sickles, causing the blood to collect in the lungs. So, anytime someone tells me about a patient with sickle cell disease, alarms go off in my head and my anxiety level increases to maximum. Having been told that this little boy had sickle cell disease and had acute chest syndrome, my heart was now in my throat. Once again, as I have seen before, I recognized that look of doom in his eyes.

He was a beautiful boy who was gasping in desperation for each breath. He was also in severe abdominal pain due to his illness. As a result of his abdominal pain, he began to breathe shallowly, triggering the oxygen levels in his lungs to drop, causing his blood cells to sickle, which resulted in his acute chest syndrome. He had a high fever, was on extremely high levels of oxygen, and was in significant respiratory distress. At this point, his only salvation would be an exchange transfusion. A simple transfusion is a process by which type-specific blood is given over a couple of hours through an IV.

An exchange transfusion, on the other hand, is a labor-intensive procedure done with the goal of removing the entire body's volume of blood and replacing it with the same volume of blood from a blood-bank donor. The goal is to remove a critical percentage of sickle cell blood and replace it with normal blood. On many occasions, this can be done with an instrument similar to a dialysis machine, but with this child, I was going to have to do it by hand and remove and transfuse nearly one and a half liters of blood. My attending had to tend to another crisis, so I was on my own now, but I knew what I had to do. In order to perform this emergency exchange, I had the task of placing an arterial line and a venous line (IV). Such procedures can be painful. However, he was in so much abdominal pain and so ill, he could barely resist me while I was placing these needles in his arm.

Sickle cell disease may be one of the most horrible diseases I have ever witnessed. Once again, it is caused by an abnormal makeup of the hemoglobin molecule in the red blood cell, so that when the red blood cell is stressed for any reason, it will sickle (hence the name sickle cell). The normal red blood cell (the cell that carries oxygen) is shaped like a donut so it can flow through the blood vessels unencumbered, but a sickle cell red blood cell is shaped like a crescent or sickle. This irregular shape doesn't allow the blood to flow properly through the small vessels in the body, called capillaries, and that creates a multitude of problems, including severe pain crises, painful inflammation of fingers and toes, infection within the bones, strokes, blood cells breaking open abnormally, the spleen enlarging and filling with blood, chronic lung and kidney damage, chronic anemia, severe infections, and acute chest syndrome.

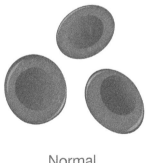

Normal
Red Blood Cell

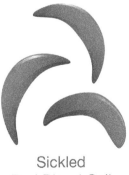

Sickled
Red Blood Cell

Acute chest syndrome is a medical emergency and can readily happen when these little guys are admitted for pain control, are placed on morphine, lie around, and don't take deep breaths. When this occurs, they can decompensate in a matter of minutes (I have seen multiple children decompensate very quickly—it always seemed to happen when I was on call—which is another reason I dislike this disease). The solution is easy—give fluids (not too much), start IV antibiotics, use morphine for pain, and for severe cases, a simple or an exchange transfusion. Needless to say, I was at his bedside most of the night caring for him and performing his exchange transfusion. His exchange took several hours while we carefully watched his blood pressure, heart rate, and electrolytes, all of which can be severely affected during this procedure. His improvement was amazingly quick after the exchange, and by morning's end, I watched a very sick little boy start to smile again and improve enough to go home the following day.

I chose to write about sickle cell because this disease affects every part of the body, and it illustrates so vividly the power of the blood. If the blood fails to perform its many tasks as described, is altered or corrupted, then pain, infection, and death results. Children used to die quite early in life from the complications of this disease. Now, with modern medicine, children are living into adulthood, yet with a whole new set of problems associated with the disease. Because of the red blood cell's abnormality, the spleen, liver, kidneys, bones, lungs, brain, and yes, even the penis, are all targets of the disease.

The pain the disease causes can be so severe that I have had morphine drips running with so much morphine it would kill two adult men. These kids experience so much pain so often, requiring frequent use of narcotics that they metabolize the drugs quickly and become tolerant. A good portion of sickle cell patients wind up as addicts due to the chronic nature of their pain and constant narcotic requirement. These kids can also grow up as adults with liver failure, hepatitis, chronic lung disease, kidney disease, and neurologic problems from recurrent strokes to name a few.

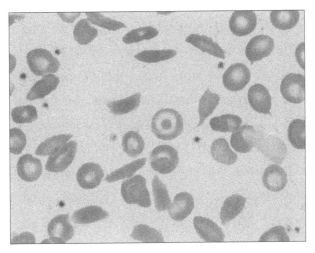

Microscopic view of blood sample with sickled cells

Thus, the *power of the blood resides in its unhindered ability to flow through the body.* So, in order for the believer to take advantage of the life-changing, strengthening, restoring, forgiving power of the blood of Christ, he must allow it to flow through him unrestricted and uncorrupted by man-made righteousness. In order for the sinner to experience the life-changing, sin-forgiving, restoring, strengthening power of the blood, he must allow Christ's blood to flow through him unrestricted. This is a very simple task, but for most is seldom done. Many Christians would rather try to correct their problems on their own, live with their sin, explain it away, or justify what and why they do what they do. They would rather spend years searching for solutions in their horoscopes, tarot cards, palm readers, psychologists, counselors, or pastors.

Some would rather try living according to an endless list of rules and regulations in an attempt to elevate a repressed conscience. As in my sickle cell patient, these are fleeting attempts designed to blunt the pain of sin and never deal with the source of the problem. The bottom line is that the believer needs to accept the propitiation that Christ made and the power that His blood has given us to survive and overcome a life born into sin (Rom. 3:23–26). The *blood—plus nothing—*is all that is needed. In other words, if our lives could be saved, healed, restored, completed, cleansed, forgiven, and unified by any other means, then Christ, God's only Son, spilled his blood in vain (Eph. 1:7–10).

We all search for power. We are always striving for more dominance or control of ourselves or others. Where is that ultimate strength or power found? Our culture is fascinated and preoccupied with hero worship. Our society also finds power in guns, cars, witchcraft, money, and muscles; which are all the wrong places. Man spends millions of dollars and countless hours trying to obtain power in cars, possessions, corporations, and political influence. In our search for strength, we spend untold time in the gym and load up on vitamins, protein drinks, creatine, and steroids. There is solar power, electric power, nuclear power, hydroelectric power, wind power, and yes, even flower power.

Power obtained in this world is easily conquered, as history has proven time and again that nothing is invincible. Samson's strength was in his hair. And when his secret was discovered, his hair was cut off along with his strength (Judg. 16:17–31). Solomon's power was found in his wisdom and knowledge; however, when he looked at life through his own wisdom (Book of Ecclesiastes), all became vain.

There is, however, unconquered power in the blood of Jesus Christ: Power to conquer the overlords of darkness, power to obtain the blessings of Abraham, power to become a joint heir in Christ, power to cleanse the darkest sin, power to heal the most broken spirit and devastating disease, power to change the most wicked heart, and power to restore the bitterest relationship.

> He has delivered us from the *power* of dark-
> ness and conveyed us into the kingdom of the
> Son of His love, in whom we have redemp-
> tion through His *blood*, the forgiveness of sins.
> (Col. 1:13–14)

There is no limit or boundaries to what the blood of Christ can do *if allowed to flow through the life* of the believer, as well as the sinner. It was shed with one ultimate purpose—to unite sinful man with a holy God. Centuries of sacrifices could never do this. His blood was shed by a cat-o'--nine-tails, it was driven into a wooden cross, and spilled by a Roman spear. How then, can that which was shed out of such intense love by a mighty God have any limit to its power?

It is so hard to understand that there is nothing that anyone can do to accomplish what the blood of Jesus did when He died on the cross. There are no works, no feats, no candle vigils, no worship formulas, and no acts of penance that can equal its power. It was the sole means by which God ordained our salvation and eternal life; it was not accomplished by human hands. Nothing else will do; there is ultimate power in the blood. "For it pleased the Father that in Him all the fullness should dwell, and by Him to reconcile all things to Himself, by Him, whether things on earth or things in heaven, having made peace through the blood of His cross (Col. 1:19–20)."

I conclude this chapter with a simple thought. There is no greater power in the blood of Christ than that of its *ability to save the lost soul*. I was a lost and lonely soul, and the blood of Jesus Christ redeemed and saved my life from a world of hurt, sorrow, and devastation. The blood set me free; and I am free indeed.

> Heavenly Father, I am sorry that I have tried to attain my salvation, my healings, and my deliverances under my own power. I am sorry I have sought selfish power through other means to fill the void in my life. I need the power of Your

blood to provide, care for, and cleanse my life. I need your strength, for mine is limited. This very moment, infuse me with the power of your blood, that is, power to change my life, power to overcome my past, power over my addictions, and power to live my life for you.

For when we were without *strength*, in due time Christ died for the ungodly. For scarcely for a righteous man will one die; yet perhaps for a good man someone would even dare to die. But God demonstrates His own love toward us, in that while we were still sinners, Christ died for us. (Rom. 5:6–8)

Have you been to Jesus for the cleansing *power*? Are you washed in the blood of the Lamb? Are you fully trusting in His grace this hour? Are you washed in the blood of the Lamb? . . . Lay aside the garments that are stained with sin, and be washed in the blood of the Lamb? There's a fountain flowing for the soul unclean, O be washed in the blood of the Lamb? Are you washed in the blood, in the soul cleansing blood of the Lamb? Are your garments spotless? Are they white as snow? Are you washed in the blood of the Lamb?"[3]

THE CELL

As darkness lurks near and blinds my eyes,

I call for help and get no reply.

As I stumble and fumble around in my cell,

I ask my way out, but no one will tell.

I walk in darkness and run into walls.

I pick myself up and take more falls.

I spin in circles looking for Light,

But the darkness, too deep to save my life.

As time ticks on, I stumble and crawl,

Hoping to live, at least until dawn.

At last, I can focus on a Light afar,

The Light I now follow, the Bright and Morning Star.

—Ike Pauli, MD

Chapter Ten

LIFE IS IN THE BLOOD

O nce again, late in the evening, I found myself on call in the NICU. As usual, when I was on call, it proved to be another sleepless night. I had just eaten a quick dinner as I hated to be away from the unit for long, given the number of ventilated and ill newborns there were in the unit. It wasn't long after I reached the NICU that I heard the loudspeaker crackle, "Dr. Pauli, pick up line one." I picked up the phone hesitantly, knowing that at this time of night it never meant good news. On the other end of the line was a neonatologist from another hospital, notifying me that he was sending us a two-hour-old baby boy who was very ill. The infant had a very aggressive resuscitation and was, for the moment, stable but wouldn't be for long.

The infant was apparently born swollen, blue, with poor respiratory effort, and poor circulation. The neonatologist continued to explain to me that the baby, after several minutes of resuscitation, was also discovered to be severely anemic. A battery of labs was subsequently sent for analysis. Ironically, up to that point, the mother's pregnancy was quite uneventful. Now, for some reason, this infant was anemic, requiring mechanical ventilation, and had begun to swell like a dry sponge in a tub full of water. I hung up the phone with a feeling of uncertainty. For a neonatologist to call me from another referring hospital meant that this baby was super-critical, and I had better be on my toes.

A few minutes later, the infant rolled through the door. From the looks of the transport team, I knew that I was in for a long night. I literally watched that baby swell before my eyes. The baby's hematocrit, which is a measure of red blood cells, was originally 8 percent when normal for a newborn was 45–60 percent. Now, after a transfusion, was raised to only 12 percent. Somehow, this baby lost nearly 90 percent of its blood volume, but there was no bleeding, placental abruption (separation of the placenta from the mother's uterus), and no evidence of hemolysis (destruction of red blood cells by the mother's immune system).

Nevertheless, the focus at hand was not why this happened, but how we were going to save this infant's life. The answer might seem simple — give him blood. The trick, though, would be to give enough blood to save his life but not so much as to overload his already-failing heart. His lack of blood had already caused a near-lethal failing heart, massive fluid in the lungs, and kidney failure.

By this time, the situation was dire, and I was very concerned that this baby would not live to see the next sunrise. I spoke with the parents and the grandparents and tried to prepare them for what may very well be a disastrous outcome. It was one of the hardest things that I ever had to do. Once again, as always, I began to pray for this precious baby and for the wisdom to care for him. Things continued from bad to worse.

We currently had limited IV access with a single umbilical cord line and were unable to secure extra IV lines due to his profound swelling, which called for assistance in placing femoral lines. We moved from dopamine drips to high-dose epinephrine to maintain his blood pressure. His lungs became so saturated with fluid that conventional ventilation was failing. It seemed that the only way to ventilate him adequately was to hand ventilate with high pressures and 100 percent oxygen. As a last resort, we were able to place him on a high-frequency ventilator, on which after hours of labor, he was finally stabilized. Thank God the on-call attending made it in to assist and guide me through the toughest hours. So far, this newborn that didn't seem to have a chance was critical but stable, and I was never so relieved when that moment arrived.

The next morning, we made rounds with our primary attending neonatologist (I felt like the cavalry had arrived) and spent an hour on his case by his bedside, making many changes to fine-tune his management. The decision was made to try surfactant (an artificial component found naturally in healthy lungs that may be lacking in severely ill or premature infants), which proved to be this child's saving grace.

By this time, I had been on my feet for twenty-four hours and I desperately needed a shower. In residency, a shower was as good as a few hours of sleep. Yet, what I needed was insignificant compared to what my tiny patient needed at that moment. It wasn't long before I noticed improvements in his condition.

Or, maybe it was the new outlook that the shower provided. Ultimately, it was an answer to prayer.

In any event, by this time, a valuable test was back, we knew why this infant was so ill and why I had spent twelve hours so intently caring for him. The Kleihauer-Betke test was positive, which meant that this child was bleeding into his mother through small microscopic leaks in the placenta. The test measures the amount of fetal red blood cells in the mother's blood. Our calculations were consistent with the test. The baby had lost between eighty and ninety percent of its red blood cells, and my attending couldn't believe it. It was a miracle this child was still alive! It would be an even greater miracle if this child survived another day.

Throughout the weeks in the NICU, he continued to improve. And after several weeks of intensive care, he came off of the ventilator and off all of his medications. To the amazement of all of our staff, this baby boy went home, normal and totally healthy in his very grateful parents' arms.

It was my second year of residency, in what would turn out to be one of the most challenging rotations of my career. There has always been a lot of mystery and dread about the months we spend in the PICU as residents during our pediatric training. The pediatric intensive care unit, in a tertiary facility like I trained in, cares for the sickest of the sick. Hospitals from hundreds of miles away and three states would send their children for us to care for them. We all know that when we are on call in the PICU, we don't get much sleep, have to be constantly on our toes, and be at the top of our game.

Tragically, because there are so many severely ill children, many times this is the pediatric resident's first experience with death. Deep down, I always knew I was destined to become a pediatrician, as I have always loved children. But all of my fears and nightmares seemed to confront me daily during my first month in the PICU. One thing, though, made me hesitate: how would I cope with the death of someone so innocent as a child? Tragically, I saw eighteen children die that month, six of those in one night. This night, my first night on call, set the tone for the month. There could never have been a worse nightmare.

It had been just a few hours into the night when we received a call that a two-year-old girl was being flown in by helicopter. She was unresponsive and intubated, after being resuscitated at a local hospital. This little girl was labeled as a "near drowning." As she rolled through the door, her respiratory pattern was one I had never seen before, only read about—agonal. It could be described like someone grunting with each breath and yet breathing with the volume and intensity of someone who had just run a marathon. It was an ominous sight. I knew this type of breathing indicated no cortical (higher brain) functioning, only brainstem activity, in other words—brain death.

Her appearance was frightening; her flaccid tone, petite size, and her cool, dusky skin left an impression on me that I will never forget. On further evaluation, her pupils were fixed and dilated; her pulses could barely be felt; and her skin mottled and clammy. We immediately secured her airway, started epinephrine, and began a cycle of fluid, blood, and platelet transfusions to maintain her circulation and keep up with the lethal processes that were going on in her body. Even for my level of training, I knew this precious child would be in the arms of Jesus by night's end, even with all of the highly-skilled and trained physicians at her side.

Her story was tragic: Her grandparents were caring for her while her mother was in the hospital giving birth to her new baby brother. The grandparents had taken her swimming at a nearby lake, turned their heads for a moment, and found her fifteen minutes later face down in two feet of water. Her heart and breathing had stopped. She was rushed to the hospital, only to be revived after thirty minutes, three rounds of epinephrine, atropine, and artificial respirations.

I watched my attending intensive care physician (one of the state's best intensivists) sit by that baby's bedside, working all night to sustain her life in spite of what appeared might be a futile act. I remember asking him, "What is the end point . . . when will we stop with what seems futile care?" His reply was simple, "When her heart stops beating." I cannot ever recall seeing an attending physician work so hard. He cared for her as if she were his own daughter.

For me, what made this horrible tragedy even more disturbing was that she looked a lot like my own little girl. She had blonde hair, big brown eyes, and was as beautiful and precious as a child could be. All that I could think about then was my own little girl. Was she safe? Was she still awake? Was she at home asleep, as she should be? Needless to say, I called home that night; I think all of us did. I just had to hear my little girl's voice. Life took on a whole new perspective that night.

We were awake all night, caring for her until I had to perform one of the most difficult tasks of my career. After her parents arrived, I placed her in her mother's arms where she took her last breath.

> Every moving thing that lives shall be food for you. I have given you all things, even as the green herbs. But you shall not eat flesh with its life, that is, its *blood*. Surely for your lifeblood I will demand a reckoning; from the hand of every beast I will require it, and from the hand of man. From the hand of every man's brother I will require the life of man. (Gen. 9:3–5)

> For the *life* of the flesh *is in the blood*, and I have given it to you upon the altar to make atonement for your souls; for it is the *blood* that makes atonement for the soul . . . for it is the *life* of all flesh. Its *blood* sustains its *life*. Therefore I said to the children of Israel, You shall not eat the blood of any flesh, for the life of all flesh is its blood. (Lev. 17:11)

In medical school, my pharmacology professor taught me three things: (1) First do no harm; (2) Oxygen is good; and (3) Blood goes around and around. The third concept sounds so simple, but it summarizes this chapter and quite possibly this book because all life is in the blood: All organs are reliant upon the blood; all tissues and cells are dependent on the blood for oxygen, nutrition, protection, communication, metabolism, elimination, and healing. To accomplish these incredible functions, the blood must constantly be circulating (going around and around). The heart pumps the blood. The kidneys filter and regulate the blood's chemistry and pressure. The liver and pancreas control the blood's metabolism. The lungs oxygenate the blood. Quite literally, all life is in the blood, and without it, life cannot exist.

As with the first baby in the chapter, who lost 80–90 percent of his blood, he demonstrated that life couldn't exist without the blood. Though we assisted in saving his life at great cost, it was a miracle he survived. In order for him to live, however, we needed to replace the blood that was lost. The second child brings home the point even more. She drowned; as a result, she died of a lack of oxygen to her tissues. Oxygen is an element the blood is designed to transport, deliver, and remove its byproduct. Once her blood became saturated with waste and was deficient in oxygen, her heart stopped. Once the blood ceased to circulate, her brain, liver, and kidneys died, leading to total body shutdown. Death of the remaining tissues of her body tragically resulted.

Jesus's shed blood is life to the heart and soul of man. In spite of all that we do or all of our attempts to become righteous or holy, we will fail without the blood of Christ. With no less importance than the physical blood flowing through our veins, the blood of Christ is the only life-sustaining substance for our spiritual lives. It washes, cleanses, protects, communicates,

LIFE IS IN THE BLOOD

provides strength, gives power, and is the sole source of forgiveness—all of which we cannot spiritually, emotionally, and intellectually live without. For man cannot live without blood in his veins, nor can he have eternal life without the blood of Jesus Christ. It is no less vital.

Why, then, did it take the blood of God's Son to give life to man? Why must there be the shedding of blood at all? First of all, man was created in the image of his Creator—God (Gen. 1:26–27). Who better then, to save the soul of man? Second, because man sinned, God would require a reckoning of his blood (being that it contained the essence of his life) (Gen. 9:5; Rom. 6:23). Without recreating the fourth through the sixth chapters of Romans and the tenth and eleventh chapters of Hebrews, I will attempt to explain, keeping in the theme of this book.

For instance, as a physician, if I saw a child dying of a fatal hemorrhage, I would first identify the source of bleeding, stop the hemorrhage of blood, give large volumes of normal saline (IV fluids) to restore blood pressure and volume, give type-specific blood if needed, and then repair the wound. I wouldn't give him a different type of blood, nor would I give him blood from a goat, sheep, or bull. Blood from an unidentified source might work briefly (temporarily) but could ultimately kill him; hence the rationale for stabilizing him with normal saline until type-specific blood could be obtained.

Likewise, in the Old Testament, God first identified our sin through the law and held us accountable by our blood (life-giving substance). He transiently provided a substitution by using the blood of animals through sacrifice. This was merely a stabilizing substitute until His perfect solution and plan could be fulfilled. He also ended the curse of death by the death of His own Son.

New life was then provided by the perfect transfusion, type-specific blood, the blood of a Man flowing from the heart of God, his Creator. The perfect solution provided by our Creator. *That solution was the final and complete act sealed with the shedding of the blood of Jesus Christ for His own creation ultimately dead in sin.* Finally, complete healing, sanctification, and restoration would then be provided through the sutures of the Holy Spirit. Where once we were forbidden to drink of the blood of animals (because all life is in the blood; Lev. 17:12), now we are commanded to partake of the blood of the Son of Man symbolically through the Holy Communion, that we may have eternal life (1 Cor. 11:25-26).

Why? All life is in the blood of Jesus Christ! It is type-specific, not for animals, angels, or demons, but for the human being. Therefore, take it and "drink ye all of it." Once again, it was a perfect transfusion provided from the heart of the Great Physician to once and for all end the power of sin and death over mankind. It was provided by the sinless Lamb of God at a specific time, with a specific purpose, and a perfect design. It cannot be explained more simply. I have listened to my pastor's sermons for nearly forty years and can hear this quote ringing in my ears and it says it all:

It was not the blood of goats and bulls sacrificed for Solomon's Temple . . . no, not that blood.

It was not the blood shed by our forefathers during the American Revolution . . . no, not that blood.

It was not the blood spilled on the sands of Norway, Korea, or Vietnam . . .

No, not that blood . . .

It was the blood shed by a Cat-of-Nine-Tails for our healing . . . That blood.

It was the blood shed through nail pierced hands on a wooden cross purchasing our redemption . . . That blood.

It was the blood that flowed from Emmanuel's veins . . . That blood.

It was the blood spilled from the side of our Risen Savior . . . The only blood that has purchased our redemption . . . That blood . . . Give Him praise!"

—John Hagee [4]

All life is in the blood!

A SINGLE CASUALTY

Driven by death . . .

In the pursuit of true life.

Caught in a conflict . . .

To end all strife.

How many have perished . . .

And how many have died?

In this Stone grinding war . . .

Fought for one life.

A battle with one casualty . . .

And only one Way to win.

A war with self . . .

Struggling to live.

A sure way out . . .

Yet, with no place to go.

Caught in the future or is it past . . .

Hashing through memories that seem so vast?

Probing for answers . . .

To end all pain.

Finding no solutions . . .

To this brutal war again.

For the casualties just seem way too high . . .

To erase the shadows in this wayward mind.

Can it be true, this blood will suffice . . .

Restoring, completely, this tattered life?

Yet, this Single Casualty provided a way . . .

That I may live . . . to see another day.

—Ike Pauli, MD

Chapter Eleven

BLOOD AND WATER

So they requested Pilate to have the legs broken and the bodies taken down. The soldiers accordingly came to the first of his fellow-victims and to the second, and broke their legs; but when they came to Jesus, they found that he was *already dead*, so they *did not break his legs*. But one of the soldiers stabbed his side with a lance, and at once there was a flow of *blood* and *water*. (John 19:31–34 NEV)

O bviously, crucifixion was not a punishment intended to bring about a quick death. It was intended to torture a man slowly while providing a powerful example to a would-be offender. Why else would a hill in plain view just outside of the city with a man raised into the sky be a chosen form of punishment? It was a slow death, intended to torture a man until he would eventually die of suffocation or hemorrhage. Apparently, the Romans, who had become quite skilled at punishing their enemies, would even offer sour wine and myrrh to provide some transient pain relief and avoid early death.

It is my understanding, from old historical accounts, that a man could stay up on a cross for days when crucified. Hence, the reason for the Jewish leaders petitioning Pilate to have those who were crucified have their legs broken, to die (and be buried) before the Sabbath and the Passover. Also, a body even though dead, might hang on a cross for days until removed as a deterrent to others for similar crimes while others would remain indefinitely. [5]

The torture lies in the mechanism of crucifixion. With nails in both hands (most likely the wrists) and feet, there would be the full weight of the man resting on the back of the cross, the nails of the hands, and the feet. In order to breathe, the victim would have to push up with his legs against the nails in the feet and pull up on the nails in his wrists. Once this agony was too great to bear, he would relax, creating more tension on his wrists and chest bearing full body weight there and would subsequently be decreasing expansion of his chest to breathe. With his lack of oxygen and drive to breathe (much like a drowning victim reaching for anything around), he would repeat the process until complete exhaustion. The victim would then die most likely of respiratory failure, infection, exsanguinations (bleeding), or dehydration.

Jesus's journey actually began in the Garden of Gethsemane where the weight of our sin, the knowledge of the imminent future, and the forces of hell were so great that He was sweating drops of blood. The amount of physical and emotional stress to cause this condition is unimaginable. Jesus later stood trial before Caiaphas once, King Herod once, and Pontius Pilate twice; yet, He was found by Herod and Pilot to be innocent of accused crimes.

Nevertheless, with the threat of riot and revolt being stirred up by a corrupt leadership (Matt. 26:59), Pilate gave Him over to the will of the Sanhedrin to bear the full measure of punishment by Roman law—scourging and crucifixion. Resultantly, Jesus was whipped with thirty-nine lashes of a cat-o'-nine-tails (a Roman whip made of lead, glass, and bone woven within leather strands, designed to rip flesh from the back of an offender), beaten, crowned with thorns, and marched through the city with a heavy cross on his back to be crucified. At some point during the journey, Simon was commissioned to carry the cross the remainder of the way (Lk. 23:26). All were extreme punishments, even in the time of Christ. This information is important in understanding why and how Jesus died on the cross.

The above account, found in John 19:34, to me, is one of the most impressive details found in the Gospels. When the Roman soldier pierced His side, he knew He was already dead—his goal was simply to make sure, as a good Roman soldier would; yet he absolutely and undeniably proclaimed it to the world. John records that blood and water flowed. When blood ceases to be circulated or agitated (due to the forces of gravity), it separates into two visible components; plasma (clear fluid) on top and blood cells (dark red) on the bottom.

If there was blood in His abdomen or chest when pierced or cut open, it would drain. If Christ had not been dead for a considerable length of time, one would probably see a bright red pulsating hemorrhage of blood. Instead, it was recorded that blood first and then water flowed. Believe it or not, multiple experiments have been performed, trying to explain the circumstances leading to Christ's death. The piercing to the left side of Christ followed by the way the blood flowed from the body, led physicians and scientists to conclude that Jesus probably died of a ruptured heart.[6]

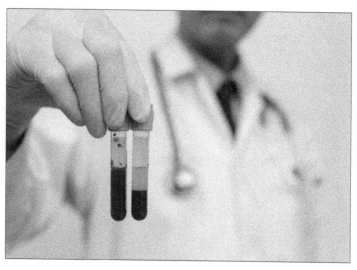

Blood in test tubes before and after being centrifuged-separating plasma and red blood cells. Note the red cells settle to the bottom

Truly, Jesus died on the cross and was dead for some time. If He had been conscious at that time or if the Roman soldiers were not certain of His death, they would have broken His legs, as the femurs of a man can contain 10 percent of the body's blood volume. Now, breaking his legs would have killed Him through internal hemorrhage and asphyxiation but may have still left room for doubt. Having blood pouring out of one's side, with this description, leaves no room for doubt even for the physician. Legs were broken, some say, because one who was crucified would no longer be able to push up on the cross to catch a breath and hence suffocate more quickly. Remember, however, that up to ten percent of the body's blood volume can be contained in the femur. It is not uncommon for someone with a single femur fracture to go into shock. Now, if both were broken, without medical intervention, one would surely die of shock, especially if crucified.

How did Jesus die then? Several vivid panoramas come to my mind as I read the Gospels. Much of this book was written before the movie, *The Passion of The Christ* was released. However, I can think of no better visual, historical, or realistic image of what happened the day of Christ's crucifixion than what was portrayed in that movie.

I have pictured a Man ushered through crowds of people and soldiers. I have imagined Him being thrown against and tied to a wooden post to be whipped with a cat-o'-nine-tails. I have seen a Man's flesh being ripped from the bone as the whip rakes across His skin. I have all too vividly imagined the amount of blood that was lost from His body as it poured from His back onto the ground from such a severe beating. It is my understanding that it was not uncommon for people to die from such a beating alone, much less in conjunction with crucifixion. (I think the movie portrayed this very graphically and vividly.)

As He was removed from the post, hunched over from pain and exhaustion, He was struck repeatedly by soldiers. He may even have been struck multiple times with blunt objects. To add insult to injury, a crown of thorns was thrust on His head with the characteristic one- to two-inch thorns burying deep in His skull.

Exhausted, humiliated, beaten, and in pain, He began to carry His cross out of the city, stumbling and falling as the weight of the cross crushed His tattered body, pinning Him to the ground while the crowd spat on His open wounds and blood-soaked body. Apparently early in the journey, a man named Simon was forced to carry the cross the remainder of the way.

I can only imagine the pain as He was laid on the cross, jagged wood upon the gaping wounds on His back. I cringe at the picture of spikes nailed through His wrists and feet and at the sound of the hammer pounding hideously large iron spikes through His body into His cross. Finally, I bow my head at the incredible pain endured as He was raised to His final destination. "So when Jesus had received the sour wine, He said, 'It is finished!' And bowing His head, he gave up his spirit (John 19:30)."

Blood and water flowed from His side when He was pierced. This means that he had free blood in His abdomen or His chest cavity. As a physician, I know the only way for this to happen would be for Him to have sustained severe chest or abdominal trauma. Possible causes would be a ruptured heart or crushing of the aorta from something very heavy—like a cross falling on Him with incredible force. Other causes could include a liver or spleen laceration from a severe beating with clubs or fists. Regardless of the mechanism, the observation of John was so insightful and specific that, quite frankly, Jesus died (and not merely swooned) on the cross from a severe beating, tortured until His last breath—all recorded with remarkable detail so that we might believe. As noted earlier, Josh McDowell in his *New Evidence that Demands a Verdict*, pp. 21–25, cites historical writings and expert accounts that confirm my clinical observations and the brutality in which Jesus was treated. These details may shed new light on the prophecies of Isaiah:

> He is despised and rejected by men, a Man of sorrows and acquainted with grief. And we hid, as it were, our faces from Him; He was despised, and we did not esteem Him. Surely He has borne our grief and carried our sorrows; yet we esteemed Him stricken, smitten by God, and afflicted. But He was wounded for our transgressions, He was bruised for our iniquities; the chastisement for our peace was upon Him, and by His stripes we are healed. (Isa. 53:3–5 NKJV)

Recently, my wife, Vicki, was going through a difficult time as we all do on occasion. She began to question God's love and asked for a Word to help her through and reaffirm His love for her. During her prayer time, God pointed her to Isaiah 49:14–16:

But Zion said, "The Lord has forsaken me, And my Lord has forgotten me." "Can a woman forget her nursing child, and not have compassion on the son of her womb? Surely they may forget, Yet I will not forget you. See, *I have inscribed you on the palms of My hands.*"

God then reminded her just how He inscribed her on His palms—with a vivid vision of nails being driven through His hands.

This is exactly the point of this chapter—to bring home the immense love that God expressed to His children by enduring the intense suffering, pain, and shame of the cross. Furthermore, to bring home the finality of what was done through the blood that was shed, He did not only allow His only Son to die, but to be beaten, humiliated, and tortured as He bore the fullness of our sin. The legions of hell surrounded Him that day and threw everything they had at Him, all to no avail. Thus, once and for all, He would provide a way for sinful man to reach a holy God. He died a gruesome death, providing atonement for a gruesome, sinful people.

Blood and water flowed from His beaten body, providing our healing. Blood and water flowed, securing our protection. Blood and water flowed, purchasing our forgiveness. Blood and water flowed, infusing us with power. Blood and water flowed to unite us with a great and holy God. Blood and water flowed to cleanse us from sin. Blood and water flowed to give us new and abundant life. Blood and water flowed to forever mark our identity. Nothing we do or say (no matter how good we may be), no formulas for worship (whether we dance, clap, or shout), and no sacrifices we make can give us access to God without the shed blood of Christ.

Rich or poor, righteous or sinner, male or female, child or adult—no one can obtain access to God without the blood of Jesus. Is this redundant? May it never be! For as Moses took the blood and sprinkled it on the people sealing their covenant with God (Ex. 24:7–8), so also God poured the blood of His Son, the New High Priest (Heb. 7:21) on all who dare to accept Him, signing the new covenant—an unbreakable bond fulfilling the reckoning for our own sin (Gen. 9:5). As such, we are made joint heirs in Christ Jesus, (Rom. 8:17) and adopted into God's family, no longer as stepchildren left to eat the leftovers. So, Christ did not come into the world and shed His blood merely that we might make it to heaven. He came to shed His blood that we might have a relationship with a holy God, live a victorious and fulfilled life, and that through that relationship with Him, Heaven would become our final home. Blood and water flowed and still flows today.

Make no mistake about it—blood and water flowed for you!

From the lyrics of Robert Lowry (1826–1899):

What can wash away my sin?

Nothing but the blood of Jesus.

What can make me whole again?

Nothing but the blood of Jesus.

Oh precious is the flow,

That makes me white as snow.

No other fount I know,

Nothing but the blood of Jesus.

For my pardon this I see,

Nothing but the blood of Jesus.

For my cleansing this my plea,

Nothing but the blood of Jesus.

This is all my hope and peace,

Nothing but the blood of Jesus.

This is all my righteousness,

Nothing but the blood of Jesus.

Chapter Twelve

NOTHING BUT THE BLOOD

I was in my third year of residency, and I was treating a very sick infant in the NICU who was born prematurely at twenty-eight weeks, weighing less than two pounds. As a result of a series of serious medical problems caused by his prematurity, the baby required numerous blood transfusions, aggressive ventilator settings, and an overwhelming number of IV medications. We could no longer draw blood from his central lines because they were all utilized, and his minuscule peripheral veins were blown from previous IV attempts.

Consequently, my tiny patient needed another blood transfusion that once again required a blood sample to type and cross-match his blood. Since our access was limited, our next course of action was an arterial stick to obtain our sample. In small infants, arterial blood draws are usually a last resort and hitting this infant's arteries was like trying to thread a needle with a piece of yarn.

Unbelievably, after only two attempts, I obtained the needed blood. As I was placing the butterfly needle into the sharps container for medical waste, it curled around and lodged deeply in my hand. I remember the thoughts racing through my mind as I pulled the deeply-embedded needle out of my hand: "Was there a lot of blood in the needle?" "How many units of blood did this infant receive?" "Could any of those units have been contaminated with HIV, hepatitis B, or Hepatitis C?" "Now I am going to have to fill out an incident report!"

I performed the necessary cleansing procedures and filled out the required paperwork in triplicate. The next morning, I went to start the six-month process of blood draws to ensure I did not contract the HIV virus. Within a few days, I discovered that the infant was HIV negative, but I still had to live with the insecurity of, "Am I contaminated?"

I nevertheless held to the promises found in God's infallible Word that declares, "No weapon that is formed against you shall prosper (Isa. 54:17 KJV). I chose not to fear, for the Lord mandates, "You shall not be afraid of the terror by night, Nor of the arrow that flies by day, Nor the pestilence that walks in darkness, nor of the destruction that lays waste at noonday (Ps. 91:5–6 NKJV)." I thank God that after multiple HIV tests later, it was confirmed that I was not infected!

Unbelievably, there was a time when surgeons felt safe to operate without gloves. Even thirty years ago, in developed countries, the worst physicians had to concern themselves with during invasive procedures was potential wound infections. Now, we are constantly living with the threat of HIV, Hepatitis B, C, and D (and nearly every other letter of the alphabet).

Physicians abroad are on the front lines of threats like AIDS, anthrax, Ebola, bird flu, and MRSA (Methicillin Resistant Staph

Aureus). In reality, some modern-day plagues have no absolute cures. Now, even bacterial disease is becoming increasingly resistant to antibiotic therapies at alarming rates. The days of the curative "penicillin shot" are over, and the days of multiple drug regimens for once seemingly simple infections are now commonplace.

For example, I recently had an infant in the hospital with E. coli sepsis that required treatment with three different antibiotics to clear his infection. Medical literature is saturated with concerns that the next decade holds no new antibiotics to battle some of our deadliest diseases because research cannot keep up with resistance of bacteria to new antibiotics.

Nevertheless, every day, physicians like me walk in the midst of disease, heartache, and death. Every day, I praise God for His protection and healing power. The Psalmist said it best: "Yea though I walk through the valley of the shadow of death, I will fear no evil (Ps. 23:4 NKJV)." In spite of the risk, the stress, and the challenges, as healthcare providers, we do our best to treat, to cure, and to control disease, all the while trying to dodge and escape its caustic clutches.

Sometimes it feels like we are running around in the middle of the street, trying to avoid being hit by a truck during rush-hour traffic. However, no matter the danger, we do our best to protect our patients and ourselves by using specialized equipment and sterile techniques.

We painstakingly double wrap and sterilize all equipment. We wear gloves, gowns, masks, and face shields in an attempt to control the spread of disease. Daily, we wash our hands, use specific sanitizers, and vaccinate to prevent infection. We even heat our instruments up to over 250 degrees to sterilize them. Some orthopedic surgeons even wear apparatuses similar to space suits during some invasive surgeries. All procedures, no matter how simple or complex, are carefully thought out and wisely executed to avoid contamination.

In spite of it all, our mission is to walk in the midst of disease, attempting to care for and cure those who are suffering from a myriad of invisible invaders. We attempt to accomplish this task by struggling to contain and avoid the reach of the attacker's deadly tentacles. It sounds dramatic, but in reality, as you have read in previous chapters, our bodies are under continuous attack from foreign invaders.

Ultimately, it is the responsibility of our body's immune system to identify, seek out, wall off, and destroy any threat that strives against it. It is also important for the very same immune system to avoid any violent reaction that would cause it to destroy *itself*. Identifying the assailant, distinguishing it from healthy cells, and retaining a permanent memory against that specific aggressor are of utmost importance as well.

If any part of our immune system's protective processes are not operating or are dysfunctional then the "invader" has a devastating advantage within any infectious battle. Bottom line: our bodies are in a constant state of war with an overwhelming number of fungi, parasites, viruses, and bacteria that have "disguised" themselves to avoid detection. What is even more frightening—many invaders, even if detected, have developed unique survival mechanisms to survive attack.

These intruders may also have specific toxins that poison the host, blunting its protective responses. Human immunodeficiency virus (HIV) is one of those stealthy viruses that rapidly mutates, making it difficult to make a vaccine. It also has a predilection for infecting the key immune cells in the body, leaving the immune system extremely compromised.

I had not thought about how this parallels the mental, emotional, and spiritual realm until I heard a message by Dr. Jim Morocco on "Defilement." His accurate contention was that the forces of darkness, principalities, and others described in Ephesians, chapter 6, are constantly engaged with us physically, emotionally, intellectually, and spiritually to infect, distract, steal, and destroy our lives. Now, I am a pretty grounded, intellectual, and rational individual not given to superstition. But I also have a profound faith and understanding of the Word of God. The remainder of this chapter needs interpretation in that light.

Life's traumas and experiences, negative words, curses pronounced, and inappropriate contacts or violence all have the potential to produce ill effects upon an unsuspecting soul. Such a revelation made me think that all of the weapons of warfare God has provided the believer are listed in Ephesians Chapter 6, and it is up to us to learn to use them and apply them as any skilled soldier or physician should (2 Tim. 2:15).

However, what about the exposed areas of our lives—the times a soldier is caught unaware or is overwhelmed by superior forces when he or she is exhausted physically, spiritually, or emotionally? Remember, the enemy is ever-present, invisible, and relentless. Worst of all, the spiritual enemy of a Christian is much like a terrorist, preying on the weak without conscience. The Adversary has no desire to fight fairly. He is constantly converting any potential good (internet, television, social media, etc.) to work his evil plan. He is covert, disguised, ruthless, and attacks without the slightest conscience of who may be in the wake of his destruction. Our bodies, minds, emotions, and spirits are all under constant threat from the invading forces that seek to destroy us—what chance do we have for survival?

Spiritually, we constantly face unseen foes as discussed in Chapter 8, "Protection in the Blood." Yet there are even more deadly foes or invaders that we are exposed to that can be just as shattering to our lives as a good dose of HIV. These attackers easily become rooted and established within us, and they can remain undetected and unrecognized, but nonetheless are incredibly virulent.

They can slip in the twilights of our dreams, through close or distant relationships, and in times of intimacy or violence. They can creep in, utilize our innermost thoughts and desires, and produce a harvest of infection, destruction, and death. Fear of rejection, envy, jealousy, resentment, bitterness, insecurity, and hate are all examples of devastating emotions (invaders) that will eventually cripple a young spirit and immature mind.

Like HIV, traumatic experiences and deviant perceptions lie seemingly dormant, multiplying in our hearts and subconscious minds until triggered, and then releasing their machinery to destroy anything in its wake. Also, like HIV, the younger you contract the illness, the more devastating the disease. While, as a physician, I can use medications, surgical procedures, or manipulations of the body to produce its healing—diseases of the mind and spirit are much more difficult to diagnose and treat.

The fact is, many psychological and emotional illnesses take years to resolve, and some may never be cured at all. After all, how can a physician look into the depths of one's heart and the innermost thoughts of the mind? How can they reach into the soul with a scalpel and excise a specific horror? Furthermore, what test or scan can reveal the hidden unconscious mind? Therapists are trained for years, honing their skills with the goals of penetrating the invisible walls their patients built, attempting to protect their fragile minds. You may be thinking, "Why all the psychobabble—what is he really talking about?"

The proven results of physical and emotional abuse are overwhelming: Alcoholic parents produce alcoholic children. Parents who abuse their children produce children who are abusers. Parents who curse produce children who curse. What is much worse is that parents who curse and abuse their children may also produce children with serious mental illness.

We see it all too often in the evening news when a peaceful demonstration suddenly becomes an uncontrollable riot after some hot-headed fool ignites the crowd into a violent brawl. I have spoken to many police officers, and they tell me that the most dangerous call is a domestic dispute between a husband and wife, whose argument gets out of hand.

They have also shared that most offenders they arrest for a sexual crime have sizeable amounts of pornography in their home and on their computer. The sad fact is that nearly every pedophile has been sexually abused at some time in their life. What is even more disturbing is that due to their deep-seated pathology, pedophiles are rarely cured.

These are but a few examples of defilement and the effects they have on all of our lives. There are less extreme examples of what defilement produces, such as someone cutting you off on the road that sends you into a rage; a rude encounter in the grocery store and you smolder all day long; finding a phone number written down in your spouse's pocket or smelling new perfume on a shirt, and you automatically think they are cheating.

Defilement can also creep in through close relationships and verbal curses. A perfect example of this occurred on one of the most important days of my life. On our wedding day, my mother showed up to the fellowship hall of the church to help Vicki's mother and sisters decorate and set up for the reception. I was still in college then, working part-time. Vicki was the only one working full-time, so we were pretty broke. There was no wedding planner, sit-down dinner, band, or dance, just a short time of cake and punch as our budget was pretty thin.

It was evident when my mother showed up to help at the church that she had been drinking. After helping the family for a few hours, she left. A while later I received a call from her and could tell she was even more drunk, crying and slurring her speech. I reminded her then that our wedding was not about her and that she was not to return to the church unless she was sober at which time she would be more than welcome to be a part of our ceremony.

After hearing my conditions, her personality of rage took over and she began to curse me and our marriage. I dare not quote the string of four-letter words that came over the phone that day lest I offend the reader, but sadly, it was nothing I had not heard before. My mother even threatened to come and disrupt our ceremony—something I could not put past her.

The threats were so concerning that we placed an usher to guard the doors to ensure that she would not crash the wedding and cause a major scene. Our wedding, in spite of it all, happened with only one distraction. Vicki's younger brother, who had been ill, locked his legs, passed out, hit his head on the communion table, sustained a severe concussion, and had to be rushed to the hospital via EMS.

When I married Vicki, I gained a godly mother and father who loved and accepted me for who I was. Vicki, however, gained a mother-in-law who would never really accept her, no matter what she did to try to show her love. Behavior that I was accustomed to was foreign to Vicki. She was not adapted to that kind of rejection and, for a time, that rejection really affected our relationship as well. Going through what we did during our wedding, I knew Vicki must have loved me. Really, who would go through that kind of drama just to get married?

One day, in the early years of our marriage, we had one of the worst fights we had ever had. Exhausted, we went to our bedroom to calm down and decompress. While we were lying there, something bizarre happened. In our 550 square foot apartment, just above our small dinner table, we hung a wooden heart-shaped crafted sign that read, "God Bless This Home." Though we had a rather heated debate that night, there were no doors slammed, no things thrown, and no physical confrontations.

Yet, as we talked about the destiny of our future together, we heard the thunderous crash of that sign, which fell off the wall. As it hit the floor, it broke into two pieces. I jumped up and ran around the corner to find the fractured sign. I carried the sign into the bedroom with one piece in each hand. Vicki and I looked at each other and became speechless.

At that moment, a clear voice in my mind said, "Your marriage has been cursed." I immediately remembered what my mom had spoken the day of my wedding. I told Vicki what I had heard, and we instantaneously prayed and broke that curse—through the power and authority of the blood of Jesus.

I would like to say that our marriage has had no difficulties since that day. Yet, quite honestly, we have had our share of challenges through the years. The miracle is that we have been lovingly and faithfully married for over thirty years, in spite of the great number of divorces in my parents' and grandparents' lives.

Allow me to share another personal experience that shows how quickly the "intruder" can come into the mind and take over. I was in the third year of medical school, and my wife was working as a manager in a retail store downtown. A cardiology convention was taking place near the store that she was managing. One day during the convention, one of the cardiologists attending the convention walked into her store. As she waited on him, during the course of conversation, my wife mentioned I was in medical school. He then remarked, "You need to watch him closely because he will use you to get him through school and leave you for some cute nurse once he graduates."

Why would a doctor, an obviously educated man, plant such a carelessly negative thought? His remark undeniably defiled my wife's thoughts with a fear that was totally unfounded in our relationship. It may very well have happened to him or someone close. Has it happened to others? Yes, but as a scientist and a trained physician, he should have had enough sense to avoid unfounded and stereotypical generalizations. Nevertheless, he injected my wife with an unfounded dose of fear. For years after, if I failed to answer a call, was late from a busy day, or had an unexpected phone call there was suspicion of another woman. My wife's mind was defiled.

Similarly, in Chapter 1, "Living with Blood," I described a few of my childhood experiences that demonstrated that the lifestyles of my parents clearly defiled me. The poor choices my parents chose to make also exposed me to a great deal of what is now called "toxic stress."

Toxic stress is a culmination of extreme negative events that produce profound negative effects on logical reasoning, emotional development, physical health, level of education, and even the kind of employment one attains. A pediatric journal concluded:

In a parallel fashion, longitudinal studies that document the long-term consequences of childhood adversity indicate that alterations in a child's ecology can have measurable effects on his or her developmental trajectory, with lifelong consequences for educational achievement, economic productivity, health status, and longevity.[7]

Since science has overwhelmingly shown that *toxic events* and stress can have profound negative and irreparable damage even to the brain's neural network, the question that arises is, "What keeps individuals like myself from succumbing to the defilement of their past?" Science can propose several potential solutions, but in my life, the only way I was able to overcome personal defilement was and is through the power of the blood of Jesus Christ. When even the toughest armor fails and our skin is pierced, the blood is there to repair, *for the Word of God declares*:

> Inasmuch then as the children have partaken of flesh and blood, He Himself likewise shared in the same, that through death He might destroy him who had the power of death, that is, the devil. (Heb. 2:14 NKJV)

When the weapons of warfare breech a soldier's armaments, the blood is there to restore. When the superficial defenses of the body are breached, the blood is there to respond.

> In Him, we have redemption through His blood,
> the forgiveness of sins, according to the riches
> of His grace which He made to abound toward
> us in all wisdom and prudence. (Eph. 1:7–8)

When life's negative experiences creep into our minds with contaminated memories, the blood of Christ is there to heal and it reminds us that:

> He has delivered us from the power of dark-
> ness and conveyed us into the kingdom of the
> Son of His love, in whom we have redemp-
> tion through His blood, the forgiveness of sins.
> (Col. 1:13–14)

When the world throws destructive insults, paralyzing inse-curities, and vile vulgarities at us, the blood of Christ is there to protect and cleanse us from *all* defilement:

> But if we walk in the light as He is in the light,
> we have fellowship with one another, and the
> blood of Jesus Christ His Son cleanses us from
> all sin. (1 John 1:7)

When the forces of evil dig up, probe, and stir up sins and bitter memories of the past, the blood of Christ is there to protect, forgive, and cleanse:

> How much more shall the blood of Christ, who through the eternal Spirit offered Himself without spot to God, cleanse your conscience from dead works to serve the living God? (Heb. 9:14–15)

The blood of Jesus Christ has a power that years of psychotherapy, counseling, or psychopharmacology does not have. I am the first to admit that medical therapies are necessary and are indicated for treatment of most illnesses. Nevertheless, the blood of Jesus is the only true and final answer for disease or illness resulting from traumatic stress, tormenting unforgiveness, extreme worry, and overwhelming fear. I have no medical studies to prove my claims, just faith, personal testimonies, and personal experience of the power of the blood of Son of God. The Good News of the Gospel testifies of that:

> To Him who loved us and washed us from our sins in His own blood and has made us kings and priests to His God and Father, to Him be glory and dominion forever and ever, Amen. (Rev. 1:5–6)

I have brought you through twelve chapters of medical science, tragedy, triumph, and personal experience to bring you to this point. Until now, you have probably never seen these "blood principles" in this light. *Now what? What do you do with all that I have shared with you?*

Obviously, information is useless unless it is applied. I request that you ask yourself the following questions:

- Do I want my life to be free from defiling memories and the negative experiences of the past?
- Do I want deliverance and healing from the past, a renewed mind, and strength and hope to face the future?

If the answer to any of these soul-searching questions is yes, then applying another Man's blood over your life is the prescription for your cure. You may think it ironic, but this restorative journey begins with a simple declaration and prayer, such as this:

Heavenly Father, I repent of the sins of my past and present. I declare that I believe in Your Son Jesus Christ. I believe His life was sacrificed for me and that His blood was shed for me. I ask to be cleansed in that blood that was shed for me for the forgiveness of sins, deliverance of my past, and the healing of my mind, body, and spirit. I believe the blood of Christ will produce in me a new life, supernatural power and protection, and eternal salvation from death, hell, punishment, and the grave.

This moment, through the blood of Christ, I forgive all who have wronged me. Now, through the blood of Jesus, I break all curses spoken against me, I break all familial curses, and I break the bondage of every past experience that negatively affects me. I now willingly receive Your total healing and complete restoration.

Heavenly Father, as I place my complete faith in You, Your Word, and Your blood for my divine healing, I repent of all that I have allowed to bind me to my past. I pledge to follow your Word, being cleansed by Your blood, for the remainder of my life. Amen.

I conclude all I have written with a prescription from my heart and from the Word of God, "Therefore if the Son makes you free, you shall be free indeed (John 8:36)." That is the true freedom bought and paid for by the precious and amazing blood of the Son of God himself, Jesus Christ.

My instruction for dosage is: Don't just read about it. Apply it to your life and the doorpost of your soul because *All Life Is in the Blood*.

REFERENCES

Chapter 6:

1. "communion," *Merriam-Webster.com*, Merriam-Webster, 2018, Web. 5 November 2018.

Chapter 9:

2. Jones, Lewis E., "There Is Power in the Blood"
3. Hoffmann, Elisha A., "Are You Washed in the Blood?"

Chapter 10:

4. Paraphrased from Sermon "Prophesy of the Passover" by John Hagee.

Chapter 11:

5. McDowell, Josh, *New Evidence that Demands a Verdict,* Vol. 1 and 2, Thomas Nelson Publishers, 1999, p. 222.
6. McDowell, Josh, *New Evidence that Demands a Verdict,* Vol. 1 and 2, Thomas Nelson Publishers, 1999, p. 221–223

Chapter 12:

7. "The Lifelong Effects of Early Childhood Adversity and Toxic Stress, *Pediatrics*, January 2012, Volume 129 / Issue 1. pp. 232–246.

ABOUT THE AUTHOR

Dr. Ike Pauli is a San Antonio native having obtained his bachelor of science in chemistry at the University of Texas, San Antonio, in 1988. He worked as a chemist until his entrance into medical school in 1990. Dr. Pauli fulfilled his lifelong dream obtaining his doctor of medicine degree in 1994 from the University of Texas Health Science Center, San Antonio. He completed his pediatric training at Children's Hospital of Wisconsin in Milwaukee, Wisconsin, in 1997. He returned to San Antonio and joined Northeast Pediatric Associates, P.A. in July of 1997. He is board certified by the American Academy of Pediatrics and is a fellow of the American Academy of Pediatrics. He has also presented his published research at local, regional, and national conferences in pediatrics. Dr. Pauli continues to serve his community in private practice at Northeast Pediatric Associates for over twenty years where he is president and CEO. Dr. Pauli is an associate clinical professor for two local medical schools, teaching and mentoring medical students in his busy office practice.

Dr. Pauli spends most of his time with his three greatest loves; his faith, his family, and his pediatric practice. He has been married for over three decades to the love of his life, Vicki, and has an amazing daughter, Paisley, who is currently attending the University of the Incarnate Word School of Medicine. He devotes a great deal of time to his church, Cornerstone, with their international television ministry for over thirty-five years, as medical director and school board president for Cornerstone Christian School for over ten years, and co-director of their mobile medical unit.

CPSIA information can be obtained
at www.ICGtesting.com
Printed in the USA
FFHW021717210219
50634957-56022FF